From Qi to Flow:

Regulate Menstrual Cycle Naturally with Traditional Chinese Medicine

Li Mei Chen

Azure Publishing Co.

From Qi to Flow: Regulate Menstrual Cycle Naturally with Traditional Chinese Medicine

by Li Mei Chen

Published by Azure Publishing Company

Copyright © 2024 by Li Mei Chen

All rights reserved. No part of this book shall be reproduced by any mechanical, photographic, or electronic process, or in the form of a phonographic recording, nor may it be stored in a retrieval system, transmitted, or otherwise be copied for public or private use---other than for "fair use" as brief quotations embodied in articles and reviews without prior written permission of the publisher.

This publication contains the opinions and ideas of its author. It is intended to provide helpful and informative material on the subject matter covered. It is sold with the understanding that the author and publisher are not engaged in rendering professional services in the book. If the reader seeks personal assistance or advice, a competent professional should be consulted.

The author of this book does not dispense medical advice nor prescribe the use of any technique as a form of treatment for physical or medical problems without the advice of a physician, either directly or indirectly. The intent of the author is only to offer information of a general nature to help the readers. The author of this book and the publisher assume no responsibility for your actions in the event you use any of the information in this book for yourself.

ISBN 9798324959937

Printed in U.S.A.

Contents

9. Integrating TCM Principles into Modern Living 97

10. Finding Your Flow: Supporting Menstrual Harmony Through Balance 103

Author's Note

In this book, organ names are written in capital letters to signify their representation within Traditional Chinese Medicine (TCM). TCM organs are conceptual entities that encompass a broader range of functions and attributes than their Western anatomical counterparts. In TCM, organs are viewed as dynamic systems that interact with each other and with the body's energy pathways (meridians) to maintain balance and harmony within the body. Writing organ names in capital letters serves as a visual cue to remind readers that these terms refer to the TCM understanding of organs, which may differ in scope and interpretation from Western anatomical terms.

Introduction:

Unveiling the Ancient Wisdom

Traditional Chinese Medicine (TCM) is a holistic system of medicine that has been practiced for thousands of years. Its roots date back over 2,000 years to ancient China, where it was developed through careful observation of natural phenomena and the human body. TCM encompasses a wide range of practices, including acupuncture, herbal medicine, dietary therapy, and exercise (such as tai chi and qigong).

The History and Evolution of TCM

Throughout its long history, TCM has evolved and adapted to the changing needs of society. Its foundations lie in the ancient texts such as the *Huangdi Neijing* (The Yellow Emperor's Inner Classic) and the *Shennong Bencaojing* (The Divine Farmer's Materia Medica), which set forth the principles of balancing the body's energy (qi), maintaining harmony between the body and mind, and promoting overall well-being.

As TCM spread across Asia, it was influenced by various cultures and regions, each contributing to its diverse and rich history. Over the centuries, TCM has been continuously refined and expanded, incorporating new techniques and knowledge.

In modern-day China and other East Asian countries, TCM continues to be an integral part of healthcare. It is often used alongside Western medicine, providing a complementary approach to treatment. Many hospitals in China offer TCM and

Western medicine services, allowing patients to benefit from
both approaches.

Scientifically Proven Efficacy

The scientific community has increasingly recognized the
potential benefits of TCM. Numerous studies have been
conducted on acupuncture and herbal medicine, demonstrating
their efficacy in treating a range of conditions, including pain,
stress, digestive issues, and gynecological disorders. For
example, acupuncture has been shown to relieve menstrual pain
and regulate the menstrual cycle in some women.

While TCM may not always align with Western medical
practices, its holistic approach and individualized treatments can
offer significant advantages in addressing the root causes of
various health issues. This makes TCM an attractive option for
an alternative or complementary treatment.

TCM for Menstrual Cycle Regulation

TCM has proven particularly effective in regulating menstrual
cycles and treating reproductive complaints such as PMS and
PCOS. It views menstrual irregularities and gynecological
conditions as imbalances within the body's systems, particularly
in the qi and blood flow.

By employing acupuncture, herbal medicine, and dietary
therapy, TCM practitioners can address these imbalances and
restore harmony within the body. For example, acupuncture can
stimulate specific points to regulate the menstrual cycle, while
herbal medicine can nourish the blood and balance hormones.

TCM's focus on individual constitution and holistic treatment
allows for personalized care tailored to each woman's unique
needs. This is a key reason why TCM was chosen as the

approach for this book—to provide comprehensive guidance on regulating menstrual cycles and healing gynecological diseases.

Modernization and Adaptation of TCM

As the world becomes more connected and technology driven, TCM has evolved to meet the demands of modern life. In China and other East Asian countries, TCM is now supported by advanced research and technology. Herbal remedies are often available in convenient forms such as capsules and granules, making them easier to incorporate into busy lifestyles.

Furthermore, TCM practices such as acupuncture and massage have been adapted to fit modern healthcare settings, with clinics offering quick and accessible treatments for common ailments. These adaptations allow TCM to be a more viable option for people with hectic schedules.

Interesting Anecdotes

One of the most intriguing aspects of TCM is its deep connection to nature and its ability to draw from the wisdom of centuries-old traditions. For example, the discovery of acupuncture points is said to have come from observing the behavior of animals that instinctively press certain parts of their bodies to relieve pain.

In recent years, TCM has gained popularity worldwide, with celebrities and athletes endorsing its benefits. This growing acceptance highlights the increasing appreciation for holistic and natural approaches to health.

Traditional Chinese Medicine offers a holistic, patient-centered approach to healthcare that focuses on achieving balance and harmony within the body. Its long history, scientific evidence, and modern adaptations make it a valuable resource for regulating menstrual cycles and healing gynecological diseases.

This book aims to provide readers with the knowledge and tools needed to integrate TCM practices into their lives, helping them achieve greater menstrual wellness and overall well-being.

1

Key Concepts of Traditional Chinese Medicine

Traditional Chinese Medicine (TCM) offers a holistic approach to health and wellness through a rich tapestry of interconnected concepts and principles. In this chapter, we will explore some of the key concepts that form the foundation of TCM, helping you understand the essence of this ancient practice and how it can guide you towards balanced and optimal health.

Jing, Qi, Shen

Jing (Essence)

Jing can be likened to the genetic material and life force in Western medicine. It is the foundational energy that supports growth, development, and reproduction. When depleted, it can lead to premature aging, fatigue, and weakened immunity. To restore Jing, nourish yourself with a balanced diet, adequate rest, and lifestyle practices that avoid overexertion.

Qi (Vital Energy)

Qi is the life force that flows through the body, governing physical and mental functions. It is similar to the concept of energy flow in Western physiology. When Qi is depleted, you may experience fatigue, weakness, and decreased immune function. Restoring Qi involves practices such as acupuncture, qigong, and dietary adjustments to promote energy flow.

Shen (Spirit)

Shen represents the mind, consciousness, and emotional well-being. It is likened to mental and emotional health in Western medicine. When depleted, it can lead to anxiety, depression, and other emotional disturbances. Restoring Shen requires practices that promote mental clarity and emotional balance, such as meditation, mindfulness, and nurturing social connections.

The Organ System in TCM Perspective

The organ systems in TCM differ in concept and function from their Western anatomical counterparts. TCM organ systems are conceptual entities that encompass not only physical organs but also related functions, emotions, and energetic qualities. For example, the Liver in TCM is not only responsible for detoxification and metabolism but also for the smooth flow of Qi (vital energy) and the regulation of emotions such as anger and frustration. Similarly, the Spleen in TCM governs digestion and nutrient absorption but also plays a role in transforming and transporting Qi and Blood throughout the body. These differences highlight the holistic approach of TCM, which views organs as dynamic systems interconnected with the body's overall energy balance.

Zang and Fu are fundamental concepts in TCM that refer to the internal organs and their functions. Zang organs are considered Yin in nature and include the Heart, Liver, Spleen, Lung, and Kidney. They are responsible for storing vital substances, such as Blood and Essence, and regulating physiological processes. Fu organs, on the other hand, are considered Yang in nature and include the Gallbladder, Stomach, Small Intestine, Large Intestine, Bladder, and Triple Burner. Fu organs are responsible for receiving and digesting food, transforming nutrients, and eliminating waste products. Understanding the roles of Zang and Fu organs is essential in TCM diagnosis and treatment, as imbalances or dysfunctions in these organs can lead to various health issues and disharmonies within the body.

Five Zang Organs

The five Zang organs are the Heart, Liver, Spleen, Lung, and Kidney. They are considered the "solid" organs and are responsible for storing essential substances and maintaining internal harmony. Zang organs are considered Yin in nature.

Heart (Xin)

The Heart governs blood circulation and houses the Shen (spirit), playing a central role in mental and emotional well-being. It controls consciousness, memory, and sleep, and influences emotional responses and cognitive functions. The Heart's energy manifests in the complexion, speech, and vitality of an individual. Imbalances in the Heart can lead to symptoms such as insomnia, palpitations, anxiety, and memory problems.

Liver (Gan)

The Liver stores blood, regulates Qi (vital energy) flow, and governs the smooth flow of emotions and Qi throughout the body. It also controls the tendons and nails, ensuring flexibility and strength. The Liver's energy influences decision-making, planning, and vision for the future. Imbalances in the Liver can manifest as anger, irritability, menstrual irregularities, headaches, and vision problems.

Spleen (Pi)

The Spleen governs digestion and transformation, extracting nutrients from food and fluids and transporting them to the body's tissues. It regulates the distribution of fluids, controls the muscles, and supports the immune system's function. The

Spleen's energy is responsible for nourishing the body, providing energy for daily activities, and promoting clear thinking. Imbalances in the Spleen can lead to symptoms such as fatigue, poor appetite, bloating, and weak muscles.

Lungs (Fei)

The Lungs govern respiration and control the circulation of Qi and Wei (defense) Qi throughout the body. They are responsible for inhaling fresh Qi and exhaling waste Qi, as well as dispersing Wei Qi to protect the body from external pathogens. The Lungs also regulate the skin's health, influence the voice, and govern the body's ability to adapt to changes in the environment. Imbalances in the Lungs can manifest as respiratory issues, skin disorders, grief, and weakened immunity.

Kidneys (Shen)

The Kidneys store Essence (Jing), govern reproduction, and regulate the body's growth, development, and aging process. They control the bones, teeth, and hair, as well as the body's water metabolism. The Kidneys also house the Zhi (willpower) and govern the innate vitality and vitality of an individual. Imbalances in the Kidneys can lead to symptoms such as low back pain, infertility, weak bones, urinary problems, and fear.

Six Fu Organs

The six Fu organs are the Small Intestine, Large Intestine, Stomach, Gallbladder, Bladder, and Triple Burner. They are considered the "hollow" organs and are responsible for processing and transporting substances. Fu organs are considered Yang in nature.

Gallbladder (Dan)

The Gallbladder stores and excretes bile, aiding in the digestion and absorption of fats. It governs decision-making, courage, and assertiveness, influencing a person's ability to make clear judgments and take decisive action. The Gallbladder's energy is responsible for strategic planning, foresight, and the ability to adapt to changing circumstances. Imbalances in the Gallbladder can manifest as gallstones, digestive issues, indecision, and timidity.

Small Intestine (Xiao Chang)

The Small Intestine receives and digests food, separating the pure from the impure and transporting nutrients to the Large Intestine for elimination. It governs discernment, clarity of thought, and the ability to make distinctions, ensuring efficient processing of information and experiences. The Small Intestine's energy also influences the absorption of nutrients on a physical and emotional level. Imbalances in the Small Intestine can lead to symptoms such as abdominal pain, diarrhea, confusion, and difficulty making decisions.

Stomach (Wei)

The Stomach receives food and fluids, breaks them down into smaller particles, and sends them to the Small Intestine for further digestion and absorption. It governs nourishment, satisfaction, and contentment, influencing an individual's ability to feel fulfilled and satisfied in life. The Stomach's energy also plays a role in mental clarity, concentration, and the ability to focus on tasks. Imbalances in the Stomach can manifest as digestive issues, poor appetite, emotional hunger, and worry.

Large Intestine (Da Chang)

The Large Intestine receives waste from the Small Intestine, absorbs water and electrolytes, and forms feces for elimination. It governs release, letting go, and the ability to eliminate physical and emotional toxins from the body. The Large Intestine's energy also influences the ability to set boundaries, establish routines, and maintain order in one's life. Imbalances in the Large Intestine can lead to symptoms such as constipation, diarrhea, bloating, and difficulty letting go of past experiences.

Urinary Bladder (Pang Guang)

The Urinary Bladder stores and excretes urine, regulating the body's fluid balance and eliminating waste products. It governs resilience, adaptability, and the ability to recover from setbacks, ensuring the body's ability to respond to challenges and maintain equilibrium. The Urinary Bladder's energy also influences sleep patterns, urinary function, and the body's ability to conserve energy. Imbalances in the Urinary Bladder can manifest as urinary issues, fatigue, emotional instability, and difficulty coping with stress.

Triple Burner (San Jiao)

The Triple Burner is a functional concept in TCM that regulates the body's metabolism and fluid distribution. It is divided into three areas—upper, middle, and lower—each responsible for specific functions related to digestion, respiration, and elimination. The Triple Burner governs communication between the internal organs, ensuring harmonious interactions and coordination of bodily functions. Imbalances in the Triple Burner can lead to symptoms such as fluid retention, digestive disturbances, and metabolic disorders.

Both the Zang and Fu organs work together to maintain balance in the body. Imbalances in these organs can lead to various health issues, so maintaining their harmony is key to overall well-being.

The Meridian System

The meridian system in TCM is a network of channels or pathways through which Qi and Blood flow throughout the body. These meridians connect the internal organs, tissues, and structures, forming a complex web of energy pathways that regulate physiological and psychological functions. There are twelve main meridians, each corresponding to a specific organ system, such as the Lung meridian, Liver meridian, and Kidney meridian. Additionally, there are eight extraordinary meridians, which play a more profound role in regulating the flow of Qi and Blood and are often used in advanced TCM treatments.

In TCM theory, each meridian is associated with specific functions, emotions, and sensations, and they are named according to the organs they traverse. For example, the Liver meridian not only influences the Liver organ but also governs the smooth flow of Qi, regulates emotions such as anger and frustration, and manifests symptoms such as headaches or menstrual irregularities when imbalanced. The meridian system serves as a framework for understanding the interconnectedness of the body's internal and external environments, as well as the dynamic relationship between physical health and emotional well-being. By assessing the flow of Qi and Blood along the meridians, TCM practitioners can identify imbalances or blockages and develop treatment strategies to restore harmony and vitality to the body.

Body Constitution

Understanding body constitution is essential in Traditional Chinese Medicine (TCM) as it helps determine an individual's unique physiological and psychological characteristics, as well as their susceptibility to certain health issues. In TCM, body constitution is viewed as the inherent balance of yin and yang energies within the body, which influences various aspects of health and well-being. Each person's constitution is determined by factors such as genetics, lifestyle, environment, and diet. By identifying their body constitution, you can make informed choices regarding diet, lifestyle, and healthcare practices to maintain balance and prevent imbalances that may lead to illness.

In TCM, there are five primary body constitution types, each characterized by different patterns of yin and yang energies:

Cold Type

Those with a cold constitution tend to feel cold easily, have pale complexions, and experience symptoms such as cold hands and feet. They may benefit from warming foods and herbs such as ginger, cinnamon, and lamb, as well as activities that promote warmth and circulation, such as moderate exercise and warm baths.

Heat Type

Those with a heat constitution often feel hot or flushed, have a red complexion, and may experience symptoms such as excessive thirst and irritability. They may benefit from cooling foods and herbs such as cucumber, mung beans, and chrysanthemum tea, as well as practices that promote relaxation and cooling, such as meditation and gentle yoga.

Dampness Type

People with a damp constitution may experience symptoms such as bloating, heaviness, and lethargy. They may benefit from foods and herbs that help clear dampness and promote digestion, such as bitter melon, barley, and lotus leaf, as well as activities that stimulate circulation and metabolism, such as brisk walking and abdominal massage.

Deficiency Type

Those with a deficiency constitution may feel tired easily, have weak immune systems, and experience symptoms such as fatigue and poor appetite. They may benefit from nourishing foods and herbs such as chicken soup, goji berries, and astragalus root, as well as practices that support rest and rejuvenation, such as adequate sleep and relaxation techniques.

Stagnation Type

People with a stagnation constitution may experience symptoms such as tension, stress, and emotional repression. They may benefit from foods and herbs that promote movement and circulation, such as turmeric, citrus fruits, and rosemary, as well as activities that encourage emotional expression and release, such as deep breathing exercises and creative pursuits.

At the end of this chapter, a body constitution questionnaire is included to help readers identify their own body constitution type, providing a valuable tool for personalized health and wellness strategies.

The Five Elements

The concept of the Five Elements in Traditional Chinese Medicine (TCM) is a fundamental framework used to understand the dynamic interplay and relationships between various aspects of nature, including the human body, emotions, seasons, and natural phenomena. These five elements—Wood, Fire, Earth, Metal, and Water—are not merely physical substances but rather symbolic representations of energetic qualities and processes. Each element is associated with specific organs, emotions, colors, flavors, and seasons, reflecting its unique characteristics and functions within the natural world.

In TCM, the Five Elements are thought to interact with one another through a cyclical and interconnected system known as the Five Element Theory or Wu Xing. This theory describes how the elements generate, control, and influence one another in a dynamic cycle of creation and transformation. For example, Wood generates Fire, Fire generates Earth, Earth generates Metal, Metal generates Water, and Water generates Wood, forming a continuous cycle of creation. Additionally, each element exerts a controlling influence on another element, maintaining balance and harmony within the system. Understanding the relationships between the Five Elements allows TCM practitioners to diagnose irregularities and disharmonies in the body and apply appropriate treatment plans to restore health and wellness.

Wood (Mu)

Representing growth, renewal, and flexibility, the Wood element governs the Liver and Gallbladder meridians in TCM. When Wood energy is in balance, we experience clarity of vision, adaptability, and the ability to plan and execute goals with ease. Imbalances in the Wood element can manifest as frustration, anger, and stagnation.

Fire (Huo)

Symbolizing passion, joy, and transformation, the Fire element corresponds to the heart, small intestine, pericardium, and Triple Burner meridians. When Fire energy is balanced, we experience warmth, connection, and vitality. Imbalances in the Fire element can lead to emotional instability, restlessness, and insomnia.

Earth (Tu)

Reflecting nurturing, stability, and nourishment, the Earth element governs the Spleen and Stomach meridians. When Earth energy is balanced, we feel grounded, centered, and emotionally stable. Imbalances in the Earth element can result in worry, overthinking, and digestive issues.

Metal (Jin)

Signifying clarity, precision, and discernment, the Metal element corresponds to the Lung and large intestine meridians. When Metal energy is balanced, we experience integrity, courage, and the ability to let go of what no longer serves us. Imbalances in the Metal element can manifest as grief, sadness, and respiratory issues.

Water (Shui)

Representing wisdom, adaptability, and resilience, the Water element governs the Kidney and bladder meridians. When Water energy is balanced, we feel calm, resourceful, and connected to our inner wisdom. Imbalances in the Water element may cause fear, insecurity, and issues with the urinary system.

By embracing the wisdom of the Five Elements and integrating these principles into your daily life, you can cultivate balance, harmony, and vitality on all levels of being. Whether through mindful awareness, nutrition, movement, self-care, or energy healing, the Five Elements offer a profound framework for achieving optimal health and well-being.

The Six Evils

The six evils are external pathogens that can invade the body and disrupt its balance. They include wind, cold, heat, dampness, dryness, and fire. When these evils invade, they can lead to illness or discomfort:

Wind

Causes sudden changes, symptoms, or movement (e.g., headaches, dizziness).

Cold

Causes contraction, stagnation, and pain (e.g., stiff joints, cold limbs).

Heat/Fire

Causes excess warmth and inflammation (e.g., fever, rashes).

Dampness

Causes heaviness and stagnation (e.g., edema, digestive issues).

Dryness

Causes dehydration and lack of moisture (e.g., dry skin, dry cough).

Summer Heat

Causes excess heat and humidity (e.g., heatstroke, dehydration).

To prevent the six evils from affecting the body, strengthen your immune system with a healthy lifestyle, including balanced nutrition, regular exercise, and stress management. Additionally, dress appropriately for the weather and avoid extreme temperatures.

Balance, and Yin and Yang

The concept of Yin and Yang represents the duality and harmony of opposing forces in the universe. Yin is associated with qualities such as coolness, stillness, and passivity, while Yang represents warmth, activity, and aggression. In TCM, health is achieved when there is a balance between Yin and Yang. An imbalance can lead to illness and discomfort.

Let's explore the concept of Yin and Yang in the perspective of TCM.

Yin represents the passive, receptive, and nourishing aspect of life force energy. It encompasses qualities such as darkness, coolness, and moisture. Yin is associated with the substances of the body, including fluids, blood, and tissues. It is essential for maintaining balance and harmony within the body, providing the foundation for growth, repair, and restoration. When Yin is deficient or imbalanced, it can lead to symptoms such as dryness, heat, and agitation, affecting various aspects of health and well-being.

Yang represents the active, dynamic, and transformative aspect of life force energy. It encompasses qualities such as warmth, brightness, and movement, and is associated with the functional aspects of the body. Metabolism, circulation, and are examples of these aspects of Yang. Yang provides the energy and motivation for growth, development, and movement, driving the body's processes and maintaining vitality. When Yang is deficient or imbalanced, it can lead to symptoms such as coldness, lethargy, and stagnation, affecting various aspects of health and well-being.

TCM emphasizes the importance of balance in all aspects of life, including physical, emotional, and mental well-being. Imbalances can lead to health issues, so maintaining equilibrium is essential for optimal health. To maintain balance, pay attention to your body's needs and adjust your lifestyle accordingly. Incorporate TCM practices such as acupuncture, herbal medicine, and dietary adjustments to restore harmony between Yin and Yang.

By understanding these key concepts of TCM, you can gain insights into your own health and well-being, allowing you to take proactive steps towards achieving balance and optimal health.

Body Constitution Questionnaire

Instructions

For each question, rate your experience on a scale of 0 to 5:

0 - Never
1 - Rarely
2 - Sometimes
3 - Often
4 - Very often
5 - Always

Physical Health & Sensations

1. I frequently feel tired or fatigued even after a full night's rest.
2. I often experience cold hands and feet.
3. I tend to perspire easily or sweat profusely.
4. I often feel overheated, especially at night.
5. I have dry skin, hair, or eyes.

Digestive Health

6. I experience bloating, gas, or discomfort after meals.
7. I frequently experience constipation or diarrhea.
8. My appetite fluctuates greatly from day to day.
9. I often feel thirsty, especially in the evening.
10. I have cravings for spicy, sweet, or salty foods.

Emotional Health & Stress

11. I am easily irritable or experience mood swings.
12. I often feel anxious or restless.
13. I tend to feel low energy or sluggish.
14. I find it difficult to relax or have trouble sleeping.

15. I experience palpitations or a racing heart.

Menstrual Health

16. I experience irregular periods or cycle changes.
17. My periods are often heavy or prolonged.
18. I often experience PMS symptoms such as cramps, bloating, or mood swings.
19. I have experienced menstrual pain that affects my daily activities.
20. I notice spotting or unusual bleeding patterns.

How to Define Your Body Type According to the Results

Once you have completed the questionnaire, tally your total score for each question. Compare your scores in the following categories to determine your dominant TCM body type. Keep in mind that many people may exhibit traits of more than one body type:

Cold Type

High scores in questions 2 and 19. You may have cold hands and feet, prefer warm environments, and experience menstrual pain. Recommendations: Focus on warming foods and drinks, such as ginger tea, and warm clothing.

Heat Type

High scores in questions 4 and 20. You may feel overheated often, experience heavy periods, or have a preference for cooler environments. Recommendations: Emphasize cooling foods, such as cucumber and peppermint tea, and maintain proper hydration.

Dampness Type

High scores in questions 6, 7, and 18. You may experience bloating, digestive issues, and PMS symptoms. Recommendations: Focus on drying foods, such as adzuki beans, and limit dairy and greasy foods.

Deficiency Type

High scores in questions 1 and 3. You may feel tired frequently and sweat easily. Recommendations: Nourish your body with nutrient-dense foods and practice gentle exercise to build stamina.

Stagnation Type

High scores in questions 11, 14, and 15. You may experience emotional distress and have trouble sleeping. Recommendations: Incorporate stress-relief practices such as meditation and exercise to improve energy flow.

Remember that these results provide a general understanding of your body type. Consulting with a qualified TCM practitioner is the best way to receive a more accurate assessment and personalized recommendations.

2

The Menstrual Cycle According to TCM

In Traditional Chinese Medicine, menstruation is viewed as a natural and cyclical process that reflects the dynamic interplay of Yin and Yang energies within the body. Menstruation is governed by the movement of Qi (vital energy) and blood through the meridians and organs, particularly the Liver, Spleen, and Kidneys. According to TCM principles, menstruation is influenced by factors such as the balance of Yin and Yang, the state of the blood, the condition of the organs, and the flow of Qi throughout the body.

During menstruation, the shedding of the endometrial lining is seen as a release of stagnant blood and Qi from the body, allowing for the renewal and regeneration of the reproductive system. Any disruptions or imbalances in the flow of Qi and blood, as well as deficiencies or excesses of Yin and Yang, can lead to menstrual irregularities and symptoms such as pain, cramping, bloating, mood swings, and fatigue. TCM diagnosis of menstrual disorders takes into account the overall pattern of disharmony within the body, including the constitution of the individual, the state of the organs, and the influence of external factors such as diet, lifestyle, and emotional stress. Treatment strategies in TCM aim to regulate the flow of Qi and blood, tonify deficiencies, disperse stagnation, and restore balance to the menstrual cycle, thereby promoting health and well-being in women.

Menstrual Cycle from the TCM Perspective

The TCM approach to the menstrual cycle is rooted in the concept of balance, where the harmonious flow of Qi and blood ensures not only the health of the reproductive system but influences the entire body. Divided into distinct phases, the menstrual cycle is a dynamic journey that mirrors the ebb and flow of Yin and Yang.

Menstrual Phase (Yin)

This phase corresponds to the shedding of the endometrial lining and is considered a Yin phase. It symbolizes a time of rest and renewal, akin to the winter season. TCM emphasizes nourishment and self-care during this phase to replenish the body's reserves.

Follicular Phase (Yang Rising)

As the menstrual phase concludes, the body transitions into the follicular phase. Yang energies begin to rise, initiating the growth of follicles in the ovaries. This phase is marked by increased activity and a surge in vitality, reflecting the spring season in TCM.

Ovulatory Phase (Peak Yang)

At the peak of the menstrual cycle, the ovulatory phase represents the height of Yang energy. This phase aligns with the summer season, characterized by warmth and fertility. TCM views this period as an opportunity for optimal conception, recognizing the heightened vitality and energy flow.

Luteal Phase (Yang Descending)

Following ovulation, Yang energies begin to descend, leading into the luteal phase. This is akin to the autumn season, signifying a time of preparation and nourishment. Adequate nourishment during this phase is essential for sustaining a potential pregnancy and supporting overall well-being.

Qi and Blood: The Vital Essence

Central to the TCM perspective on the menstrual cycle is the concept of Qi and blood. Qi, the vital life force, provides the energy necessary for all physiological processes, while blood, nourished by Qi, is fundamental for menstruation and fertility.

Qi Flow

Smooth and balanced Qi flow is crucial for a healthy menstrual cycle. Any disruptions or stagnation in Qi can lead to irregularities, manifesting as pain, bloating, or changes in menstrual flow.

Blood Circulation

Adequate blood circulation is vital for a healthy menstrual cycle. Blood stasis or deficiency can result in various menstrual disorders, highlighting the importance of nourishing blood through proper nutrition and lifestyle practices.

The Role of Kidney Essence (Jing)

The Kidneys, according to TCM, play a pivotal role in reproductive health. Kidney Essence, or Jing, is considered the root of life and directly influences the menstrual cycle. Nourishing Jing through lifestyle choices and herbal remedies is a key aspect of TCM approaches to menstrual wellness.

The Monthly Rhythm: A Symphony of Balance

In essence, the menstrual cycle according to TCM is a symphony of balance, where the orchestrated movements of Yin and Yang,

Qi and blood, and Kidney Essence harmonize to create a beautiful and intricate dance. Understanding this rhythm allows women to attune themselves to the cyclical nature of their bodies, fostering a deeper connection with their reproductive health.

In the chapters to follow, we will explore how TCM principles guide women in each phase of the menstrual cycle, offering practical insights and strategies to enhance well-being, regulate the cycle, and promote overall vitality. As we navigate the intricate terrain of the menstrual cycle through the lens of TCM, let us embrace the wisdom that empowers women to cultivate optimal health and balance in every phase of life.

3

Fertility and Reproductive Health

Fertility and reproductive health are vital aspects of a woman's well-being, and Traditional Chinese Medicine (TCM) offers a holistic approach to enhancing these areas. In this chapter, we will explore fertility, conception, pregnancy, and feminine reproductive health from the TCM perspective. Additionally, we will provide practical TCM rituals and practices that can improve the chances of conception, taking into account individual body constitutions.

Fertility and Reproductive Health According to TCM

In TCM, fertility and reproductive health are closely linked to the balance and harmony of the body's internal systems. The concept of **Jing (Essence)** plays a significant role in reproductive health, as it governs growth, development, and reproduction. **Qi (Vital Energy)** also plays a crucial role in maintaining hormonal balance and supporting the reproductive organs.

In Western medicine, fertility is primarily understood in terms of hormonal regulation and the function of the reproductive organs.

Conception is seen as a result of a successful interaction between sperm and egg, leading to pregnancy. Pregnancy is then managed through regular medical check-ups to monitor the health of both the mother and the developing fetus.

In TCM, fertility is viewed through the lens of balance and harmony within the body, including the interaction of the **Five Elements** (Wood, Fire, Earth, Metal, and Water) and the **Five Zang and Six Fu Organs** (the solid and hollow organs, respectively). TCM practitioners aim to identify and correct any imbalances that may be hindering fertility or reproductive health.

Infertility

Infertility, defined as the inability to conceive after one year of unprotected intercourse, is a complex and emotionally challenging issue that affects millions of couples worldwide. In TCM, infertility is viewed through the lens of holistic health, considering the interplay of various factors such as Qi (vital energy), blood, Yin and Yang, and the harmony of the organ systems. Understanding the causes of infertility from a TCM perspective can provide valuable insights into treatment strategies aimed at restoring balance and optimizing fertility.

Causes of Infertility According to TCM

Qi and Blood Deficiency

In TCM, Qi and blood are essential for nourishing the reproductive organs and supporting fertility. Deficiencies in Qi and blood may arise due to factors such as chronic stress, poor diet, overwork, or excessive physical exertion. When Qi and blood are deficient, there may be insufficient nourishment of the uterus and ovaries, leading to difficulties in conception.

Yin and Yang Imbalance:
Balance between Yin and Yang is crucial for reproductive health
in TCM. Yin represents the nourishing, receptive aspect, while
Yang represents the active, transformative aspect. Imbalances in
Yin and Yang can disrupt the menstrual cycle, ovulation, and the
implantation of a fertilized embryo. Factors such as excessive
heat or cold, emotional stress, and lifestyle habits can disturb the
Yin-Yang equilibrium and contribute to infertility.

Liver Qi Stagnation:
The Liver plays a vital role in the smooth flow of Qi and blood
throughout the body, including the reproductive system. When
Liver Qi becomes stagnant due to emotional stress, frustration,
or unresolved anger, it can lead to blockages in the flow of
energy and blood to the uterus and ovaries. Liver Qi stagnation
may manifest as irregular menstrual cycles, ovulatory disorders,
or difficulty in conceiving.

Kidney Deficiency:
The Kidneys are considered the foundation of Yin and Yang in
TCM and play a crucial role in reproductive health. Kidney
deficiency, which can be either Yin or Yang deficiency, may
result from constitutional factors, aging, chronic illness, or
excessive sexual activity. Kidney deficiency can lead to
hormonal imbalances, poor egg quality, and impaired sperm
production, all of which contribute to infertility.

Phlegm-Dampness Accumulation:
Phlegm-Dampness accumulation refers to the buildup of
pathogenic fluids in the body, which can obstruct the flow of Qi
and blood and impair reproductive function. Factors such as poor
diet, excessive consumption of greasy or sweet foods, and a
sedentary lifestyle can contribute to the formation of Phlegm-
Dampness. Phlegm-Dampness accumulation may manifest as
polycystic ovary syndrome (PCOS), endometriosis, or blocked
fallopian tubes, all of which can hinder conception.

Miscarriage

Miscarriage, the loss of a pregnancy before the 20th week, is a deeply distressing experience that affects many couples on their journey to parenthood. In TCM, miscarriage is viewed as a disruption of the body's natural harmony and balance, often stemming from underlying imbalances in Qi, blood, Yin and Yang, and the organ systems. Understanding the causes of miscarriage from a TCM perspective can provide valuable insights into prevention strategies and supportive care for couples experiencing this heartbreaking loss.

Causes of Miscarriage According to TCM

Blood Stasis
Blood stasis, or stagnation of blood flow, is considered a common cause of miscarriage in TCM. Factors such as trauma, emotional stress, or chronic illness can lead to the formation of blood stasis, which may obstruct the flow of Qi and blood to the uterus and disrupt the implantation of a fertilized embryo. Blood stasis may manifest as abdominal pain, clotting during menstruation, or dark, purplish menstrual blood.

Kidney Deficiency
Kidney deficiency, particularly Kidney Yang deficiency, is associated with an increased risk of miscarriage in TCM. Kidney Yang deficiency may result from factors such as aging, chronic illness, or excessive sexual activity, leading to weakness in the uterine lining and impaired ability to support a developing embryo. Symptoms of Kidney Yang deficiency may include cold intolerance, fatigue, and lower back pain.

Liver Qi Stagnation
Liver Qi stagnation, characterized by emotional stress, frustration, or unresolved anger, can contribute to miscarriage in TCM. Liver Qi stagnation may disrupt the smooth flow of Qi

and blood to the uterus, leading to irregular menstrual cycles, hormonal imbalances, and increased susceptibility to miscarriage. Emotional symptoms such as irritability, mood swings, and depression often accompany Liver Qi stagnation.

Spleen Qi Deficiency

Spleen Qi deficiency, which may result from poor diet, chronic stress, or overwork, is another common cause of miscarriage in TCM. Spleen Qi deficiency impairs the body's ability to nourish and support pregnancy, leading to weakness in the uterine environment and increased vulnerability to miscarriage. Symptoms of Spleen Qi deficiency may include fatigue, poor appetite, bloating, and loose stools.

Heart Blood Deficiency

Heart Blood deficiency, characterized by insufficient nourishment of the Heart and Blood, can contribute to miscarriage in TCM. Factors such as chronic illness, poor diet, or emotional disturbances can deplete Heart Blood, leading to palpitations, anxiety, and insomnia, as well as increased risk of miscarriage. Heart Blood deficiency may manifest as pale complexion, palpitations, and restless sleep.

Recommended TCM Modalities for Women Planning to Conceive

TCM offers a variety of rituals and practices that can improve the chances of pregnancy by promoting balance and harmony in the body. These modalities may vary depending on the woman's body constitution and specific imbalances.

Herbal Medicine

Customized herbal formulas are often prescribed to address specific imbalances and support reproductive health. Common formulas include **Si Wu Tang**, which nourishes the blood, and **Ba Zhen Tang**, which tonifies Qi and blood.

Acupuncture and Acupressure

Acupuncture can regulate hormonal imbalances, improve blood flow to the reproductive organs, and support overall well-being. Specific acupoints are often targeted to enhance fertility.

How to self-apply acupressure

Sit comfortably and apply firm pressure with your thumb or index finger to the intended acupressure point 50 to 100 times, or for 1 to 2 minutes and release.d

Acupressure points for enhancing fertility

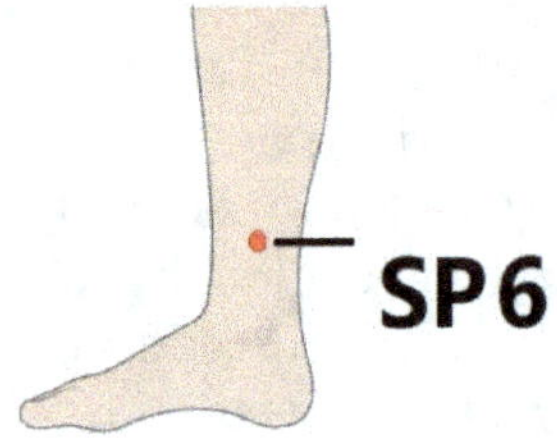

Spleen 6 (SP 6)

- Located on the inner side of the lower leg, about four finger widths above the inner ankle bone
- Regulates the menstrual cycle. Promotes fertility.

Conception Vessel 4 (CV 4)

- Located on the midline of the abdomen, about three finger widths below the navel.
- Tonifies the Kidneys and promotes fertility.

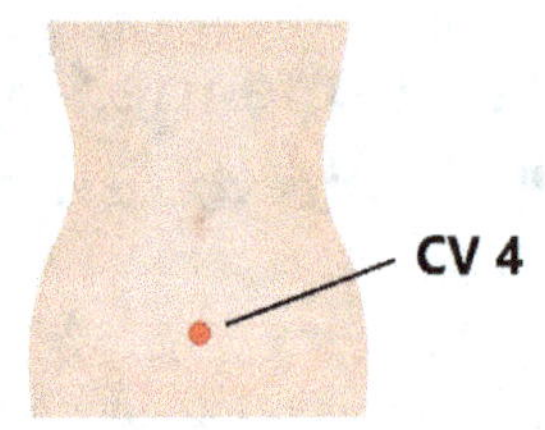

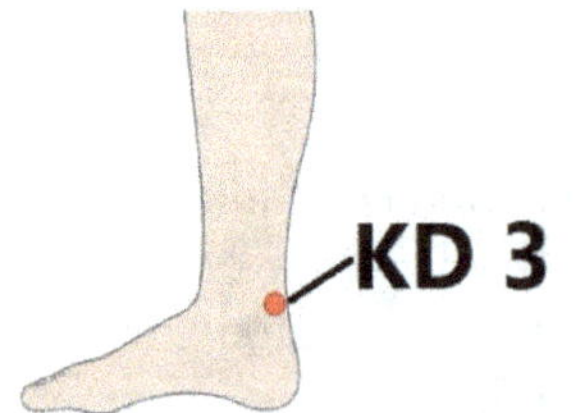

Kidney 3 (KD 3):

- Located on the inner side of the ankle, in the depression between the Achilles tendon and the ankle bone.
- Tonifies Kidney Qi and supports reproductive health.

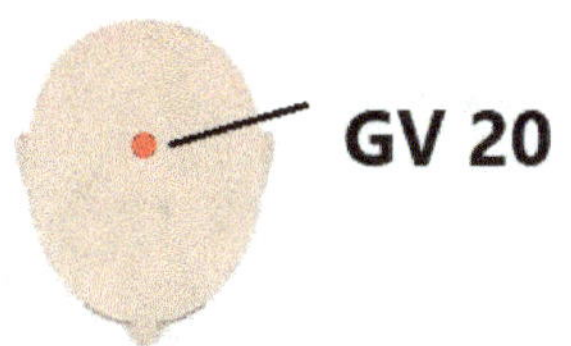

Governing Vessel 20 (GV 20):

- Located at the top of the head, in the center of the scalp.
- Calms the mind, reduces stress, and regulates hormonal balance.

Liver 3 (LV 3):

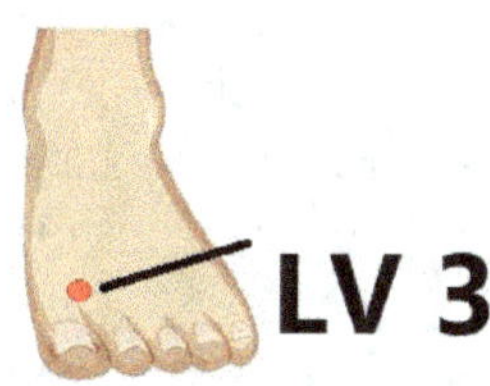

- Located on the top of the foot, in the hollow between the big toe and the second toe.
- Soothes Liver Qi stagnation and regulates the menstrual cycle.

Dietary Adjustments

A diet tailored to the woman's body constitution can support reproductive health. For example, women with a cold constitution may benefit from warming foods like spices, chicken and beef, while those with a hot constitution may benefit from cooling foods, such as watery vegetables and fruits.

Exercise and Movement

Gentle exercises such as qigong and tai chi can promote the flow of Qi and blood, helping to balance the body and prepare it for conception.

Stress Management

Managing stress through practices such as meditation, mindfulness, and yoga can help regulate hormonal balance and support overall health.

Self-Care Rituals

Incorporating the following self-care practices to improve blood flow and support the reproductive organs:

- Abdominal massages with carrier oils
- Warm compresses
- Foot soaks with salts

Lifestyle Adjustments

- Avoiding exposure to environmental toxins (i.e. minimizing exposure to plastic goods)
- Maintaining a healthy weight
- Ensuring adequate sleep

When planning to conceive, it's important for women to work with a qualified TCM practitioner who can assess their body constitution and recommend personalized practices. By integrating these TCM rituals and practices into their daily lives, women can enhance their chances of conception and support their overall reproductive health.

4

Common Menstrual Irregularities and TCM Diagnoses

When navigating Traditional Chinese Medicine in the context of women's health, it's crucial to understand how TCM views and addresses common menstrual irregularities, often described in Western medicine terms. The intricate web of TCM pathology provides unique insights into the underlying imbalances contributing to these symptoms.

Types of Menstrual Irregularities

Menstrual Pain (Dysmenorrhea) *Blood Stasis and Qi Stagnation*

In Western medicine, menstrual pain is often labeled as dysmenorrhea. TCM identifies this discomfort as a manifestation of blood stasis and Qi stagnation. When the flow of Qi and blood is obstructed, it results in pain and cramping. TCM treatments aim to invigorate blood circulation and smooth Qi flow, often employing acupuncture, herbal remedies, and lifestyle adjustments.

Irregular Menstrual Cycles *Qi and Blood Deficiency or Stagnation*
Irregular menstrual cycles, marked by variations in cycle length, may be linked to deficiencies or stagnation of Qi and blood. TCM seeks to identify the root cause, addressing deficiencies through nourishing herbs and promoting circulation to resolve stagnation. Lifestyle modifications, including stress reduction and balanced nutrition, play a pivotal role in restoring harmony.

Heavy Menstrual Flow (Menorrhagia) *Heat and Blood Heat*
Menorrhagia, characterized by excessive menstrual bleeding, aligns with TCM's concept of heat and blood heat. Excessive heat in the body can lead to increased blood flow. TCM treatments focus on clearing heat, nourishing Yin, and balancing blood to alleviate this symptom. Herbal formulas and dietary adjustments form integral parts of the TCM approach.

Scanty Menstrual Flow (Oligomenorrhea) *Blood Deficiency and Cold*
Oligomenorrhea, or scanty menstrual flow, is often associated with blood deficiency and cold in TCM. A lack of nourishment and warmth can impede the smooth flow of blood. TCM strategies involve tonifying blood, warming the body, and promoting circulation to address this imbalance.

Absent Menstrual Periods (Amenorrhea) *Qi and Blood Deficiency or Stagnation*
Amenorrhea, the absence of menstrual periods, may be attributed to Qi and blood deficiencies or stagnation. TCM treatments aim to tonify Qi, nourish blood, and address any underlying imbalances that may hinder the regular flow of menstrual cycles.

Premenstrual Syndrome (PMS) *Liver Qi Stagnation and Blood Stasis*

PMS, characterized by emotional and physical symptoms preceding menstruation, aligns with TCM's understanding of Liver Qi stagnation and blood stasis. TCM interventions focus on promoting the smooth flow of Liver Qi and alleviating blood stasis, often incorporating acupuncture, herbal remedies, and lifestyle adjustments.

Endometriosis *Blood Stasis Resulted from Qi and Blood Imbalances*

From the Traditional Chinese Medicine (TCM) perspective, endometriosis is often seen as a result of imbalances in the body's Qi and Blood. This can lead to blood stasis, which causes the blood to flow irregularly and pool in certain areas, resulting in pain and inflammation. The underlying causes of these imbalances may include emotional stress, cold accumulation, or dampness in the body, affecting the smooth flow of Qi and Blood. TCM practitioners aim to treat endometriosis by promoting the free flow of Qi and Blood, warming the body, and addressing any dampness or cold that may be contributing to the condition. This is often achieved through acupuncture, herbal medicine, dietary adjustments, and lifestyle modifications tailored to the individual's specific constitution and symptoms.

Fibroids *Blood Stasis, Liver Qi Stagnation and Accumulation of Dampness*

Fibroids are typically seen as a manifestation of imbalances in the body's Qi and Blood flow, as well as stagnation of these vital substances in the pelvic area. The condition is often linked to patterns of Blood stasis, Liver Qi stagnation, or Dampness accumulation in the body. Blood stasis can lead to the formation of masses like fibroids, while Liver Qi stagnation can exacerbate the growth of fibroids by disrupting the flow of Qi and Blood. Dampness can further contribute to the development of fibroids by causing sluggish circulation and fluid retention. TCM treatment focuses on resolving these imbalances through acupuncture, herbal medicine, and dietary modifications to regulate Qi and Blood, clear stagnation, and eliminate excess dampness. This approach aims to shrink fibroids, relieve symptoms, and restore overall balance and health.

Polycistic Ovarian Syndrome (PCOS) *Kidney Yin & Spleen Dificiency, Liver Qi Stagnation*
Polycystic Ovary Syndrome (PCOS) is understood as a complex condition resulting from imbalances in the body, particularly involving the **Kidney, Spleen,** and **Liver** organs. PCOS may be diagnosed in TCM as a combination of symptoms such as irregular menstrual cycles, excessive hair growth, and difficulty conceiving. These symptoms are linked to patterns of **Kidney Yin deficiency, Spleen Qi deficiency**, and **Liver Qi stagnation**. The Kidney's role in regulating reproductive hormones is crucial, while the Spleen's role in processing and transforming food into energy is also essential. Liver Qi stagnation can lead to hormonal imbalances and the formation of cysts on the ovaries. TCM practitioners treat PCOS by addressing these underlying imbalances with customized herbal formulas, acupuncture, dietary changes, and stress management techniques. This holistic approach aims to regulate the menstrual cycle, support hormone balance, and improve overall well-being.

Holistic Diagnosis in TCM

It's essential to note that TCM doesn't compartmentalize symptoms but considers them as interconnected manifestations of underlying imbalances. Practitioners conduct a thorough diagnosis, considering the patient's constitution, lifestyle, and emotional well-being. The holistic approach of TCM aims not only to alleviate symptoms but to restore overall balance, fostering lasting well-being.

In the subsequent chapters, we will delve deeper into specific TCM interventions and lifestyle practices tailored to address these menstrual irregularities, providing a comprehensive guide for women seeking health and vitality in their lives. As we navigate the intricacies of TCM pathology, let us embrace the holistic wisdom that empowers women to understand and cultivate balance in every phase of their menstrual journey.

5

Herbal Remedies for Menstrual Health

In the realm of Traditional Chinese Medicine (TCM), herbal remedies play an important role in promoting menstrual health and restoring balance to the body. Before delving into specific herbs used for this purpose, it's essential to understand the concept of temperature characteristics in TCM. This concept forms the foundation for selecting herbs that align with the body's constitution and imbalances.

Temperature (Energetic) Characteristics of Herbs in TCM

In TCM, herbs are classified based on their temperature characteristics, which encompass their innate energetic properties and effects on the body's balance of Yin and Yang. Understanding these characteristics allows TCM practitioners to tailor herbal formulations to address specific imbalances.

Warm herbs are often used to tonify Yang or dispel cold, while cool or cold herbs are employed to nourish Yin or clear excess heat. The combination of these herbs in formulas aims to restore harmony and address specific imbalances contributing to menstrual irregularities. Always consult with a qualified TCM practitioner to ensure the proper use and dosage of these herbs based on individual health conditions.

Hot (Yang): Hot herbs have warming properties and are used to dispel coldness and promote circulation. They are often prescribed for conditions characterized by coldness and stagnation, such as cold-type dysmenorrhea. Examples of hot herbs include ginger, cinnamon, and chili peppers.

Warm (Yang): Warm herbs also possess heating properties but are milder in nature compared to hot herbs. They help to tonify Qi and Yang energy and are often used to address deficiencies and weakness. Examples of warm herbs include Chinese dates, ginseng, and fennel seeds.

Cool (Yin): Cool herbs have a cooling effect on the body and are used to clear heat and reduce inflammation. They are beneficial for conditions marked by excessive heat, such as heavy menstrual bleeding due to blood heat. Examples of cool herbs include mint, dandelion, and mung beans.

Cold (Yin): Cold herbs have strong cooling properties and are used to clear heat and reduce fever. They are often prescribed for conditions characterized by excess heat and inflammation, such as hot flashes and irritability during PMS. Examples of cold herbs include watermelon, cucumber, and bamboo shoots.

Herbal Remedies for Menstrual Health

Herbal medicine plays a central role in TCM treatments aimed at harmonizing menstrual cycles, addressing irregularities, and alleviating associated symptoms. A diverse array of herbs are being used in TCM to bring the body, mind and spirit back into balance and harmony. The herbs chosen for TCM herbal remedies possess unique properties and therapeutic actions that target specific imbalances within the body. By understanding the characteristics and functions of these herbs, we can appreciate their profound impact on restoring balance and promoting optimal health. From tonifying blood to dispersing stagnation, these herbs offer a holistic approach to menstrual regulation that honors the intricate interplay of Qi, blood, Yin, and Yang within the body. Through the exploration of these botanical allies, you can begin on a journey towards reclaiming menstrual harmony and vitality in alignment with the principles of TCM.

❖ Types of Herbs Used in TCM

Dang Gui *Angelica sinensis, Chinese Angelica Root*
Dang Gui is a warm herb renowned for its ability to tonify blood and regulate menstruation. It is commonly used to alleviate menstrual pain, irregular periods, and blood deficiency.

Bai Shao *Paeonia lactiflora, White Peony Root*
Bai Shao is a cool herb that nourishes blood and soothes the Liver. It is often prescribed for conditions such as PMS and irregular menstruation due to Liver Qi stagnation.

Chuan Xiong *Ligusticum chuanxiong, Sichuan Lovage Rhizome*
Chuan Xiong is a warm herb that invigorates blood circulation and dispels blood stasis. It is frequently used to alleviate menstrual pain and promote the smooth flow of Qi and blood.

Gui Zhi *Cinnamomum cassia, Cinnamon*
Gui Zhi is a hot herb that warms the body and promotes circulation. It is commonly used in formulas for cold-type dysmenorrhea and irregular menstruation associated with coldness.

Mu Dan Pi *Paeonia suffruticosa, Tree Peony Bark*
Mu Dan Pi is a cool herb that clears heat and cools the blood. It is often included in formulas for heavy menstrual bleeding and inflammatory conditions of the reproductive system.

Ai Ye *Artemisia argyi, Mugwort*

Mugwort is a key herb in TCM known for its ability to warm the uterus, regulate menstrual cycles, and alleviate menstrual cramps. It is believed to promote circulation and dispel cold from the pelvic region.

Yi Mu Cao *Leonurus japonicus, Chinese Motherwort*

Yi Mu Cao is recognized for its ability to regulate menstruation and invigorate Qi. Often used in formulas for irregular periods and conditions related to Qi deficiency.

Sheng Di Huang *Rehmannia glutinosa, Chinese Foxglove Root*

Sheng Di Huang is valued for its ability to nourish yin and cool excess heat in the blood. It is often recommended for heavy menstrual bleeding and conditions associated with blood heat. It can be easily found in formulations created to address menorrhagia, irregular menstruation, and other symptoms related to heat in TCM diagnosis.

Nu Zhen Zi *Ligustrum lucidum, Privet Fruit*

Nu Zhen Zi is a cool herb frequently used to address conditions of blood deficiency and Yin deficiency that is known for its capacity to nourish both Liver and Kidney Yin. It is often included in formulas for irregular menstruation, amenorrhea, and conditions associated with kidney Yin deficiency.

Ginger *Zingiber Officinate*

Ginger is a commonly used herb for TCM decoctions, known for its warming and stimulating properties. It is an herb that can help invigorate blood circulation and support digestive health. This property makes it particularly beneficial for alleviating menstrual cramps and irregular periods by promoting smooth blood flow and reducing stagnation. Ginger can also help with nausea, which is useful for women experiencing morning sickness during pregnancy. Its anti-inflammatory and antimicrobial properties can support overall health and immunity. In TCM, ginger is often used in combination with other herbs to enhance its effects and provide comprehensive support for the formula.

While some of these herbs may not be as readily available in North America and Europe, they can often be found in specialized health food stores, herbal apothecaries, or online retailers that specialize in TCM herbs and remedies. It's important to source high-quality herbs from reputable suppliers to ensure their safety and efficacy.

❖ TCM Herbal Decoctions

Herbal remedies in TCM are typically administered as part of a comprehensive treatment plan, often in the form of decoctions, pills, or teas. However, certain herbs can also be incorporated into everyday cooking and diet to support menstrual health. For example, adding ginger to soups or stir-fries can help warm the body and promote circulation, while mint tea can help cool and soothe during times of menstrual discomfort.

In this segment, we will delve deeper into specific herbal formulations and their applications for addressing common menstrual irregularities. By harnessing the power of herbal medicine in conjunction with lifestyle adjustments and holistic practices, all women can nurture balance and vitality in their menstrual cycles, paving the way for optimal reproductive health and well-being.

Creating herbal formulations in Traditional Chinese Medicine (TCM) involves precise measurements and specific preparation methods. However, it's crucial to note that these formulations are typically prescribed by trained TCM practitioners based on an individual's specific health condition and constitution. Self-prescribing or using herbal remedies without proper guidance may lead to unintended consequences. The following are general outlines of the mentioned herbal combinations. Consult with a qualified TCM practitioner for decoctions that are tailored for your specific needs.

Here are a few notable TCM herbal combinations:

Four Substance Decoction (Si Wu Tang)

Ingredients

- 9 grams of **Dang Gui** (Angelica sinensis)
- 9 grams of **Chuan Xiong** (Ligusticum chuanxiong)
- 12 grams of **Bai Shao** (Paeonia lactiflora)
- 12 grams of **Shu Di Huang** (Rehmannia glutinosa)

Instructions Combine the ingredients in a pot with 500 mL of water. Bring to a boil, then simmer for 20-30 minutes. Strain and drink the decoction.

Application Si Wu Tang is used to regulate menstrual cycles and nourish the blood. It can treat symptoms such as irregular periods, painful menstruation, and low energy levels. The formula balances and supports the Qi and Blood, promoting smooth flow and alleviating stagnation.

Si Wu Tang is one of the oldest and most well-known herbal formulas in TCM, first introduced in the ancient text "Essential Prescriptions from the Golden Cabinet" (Jin Gui Yao Lue) around the year 220 AD. This formula is renowned for its ability to tonify blood, regulate menstruation, and nourish the Liver and Kidneys. Considered gentle yet effective, it is suitable for, and benefits people of all body constitution types. The combinations of herbs for Si Wu Tang are so versatile and adaptable that it serves as the basis for numerous TCM formulas, demonstrating its enduring utility and effectiveness in treating a wide range of health conditions related to blood deficiency and menstrual irregularities.

Cinnamon Twig and Poria Decoction (Gui Zhi Fu Ling Tang)

Ingredients

- 9 grams of **Gui Zhi** (Cinnamon twig)
- 9 grams of **Fu Ling** (Poria)
- 12 grams of **Mu Dan Pi** (Paeonia suffruticosa)
- 12 grams of **Chi Shao** (Red peony root)
- 9 grams of **Tao Ren** (Peach kernel)

Instructions Combine the ingredients in a pot with 500 mL of water. Bring to a boil, then simmer for 20-30 minutes. Strain and drink the decoction.

Application Gui Zhi Fu Ling Wan is used to treat symptoms such as irregular menstruation, uterine fibroids, and endometriosis. It helps to invigorate blood circulation, remove blood stasis, and promote the elimination of excess fluid.

Eight Treasures Decoction (Ba Zhen Tang)

Ingredients

- 9 grams of **Dang Gui** (Angelica sinensis)
- 9 grams of **Shu Di Huang** (Rehmannia glutinosa)
- 12 grams of **Bai Shao** (Paeonia lactiflora)
- 12 grams of **Chuan Xiong** (Ligusticum chuanxiong)
- 12 grams of **Ren Shen** (Ginseng)
- 12 grams of **Bai Zhu** (Atractylodes macrocephala)
- 9 grams of **Fu Ling** (Poria)
- 9 grams of **Gan Cao** (Licorice)

Instructions Combine the ingredients in a pot with 500 mL of water. Bring to a boil, then simmer for 20-30 minutes. Strain and drink the decoction.

Application Ba Zhen Tang is used to tonify Qi and blood, making it effective for women with irregular periods, fatigue, and anemia. It promotes the general health of the reproductive system.

Eight Treasures Decoction with Yi Mu Cao (Ba Zhen Yi Mu Tang)

Ingredients

- 10 grams of **Dang Gui** (Angelica sinensis)
- 10 grams of **Bai Shao** (Paeonia lactiflora)
- 10 grams of **Chuan Xiong** (Ligusticum chuanxiong)
- 10 grams of **Shu Di Huang** (Rehmannia glutinosa)
- 10 grams of **Bai Zhu** (Atractylodes macrocephala)
- 10 grams of **Fu Ling** (Poria)
- 5 grams of **Gan Cao** (Licorice)
- 10 grams of **Yi Mu Cao** (Leonurus japonicus)

Instructions Combine the ingredients in a pot with 500 mL of water. Bring to a boil, then simmer for 20-30 minutes. Strain and drink the decoction.

Application Ba Zhen Yi Mu Tang is a classic TCM herbal formula that is particularly beneficial for menstrual irregularities, blood stagnation, and Qi deficiency. This decoction with warming nature nourishes the blood and tonifies the Qi, while also invigorating blood circulation and removing stagnation, particularly in the uterus. It may help alleviate symptoms such as irregular periods, amenorrhea, and dysmenorrhea.

Six Flavor Rehmannia Decoction (Liu Wei Di Huang Tang)

Ingredients

- 12 grams of **Shu Di Huang** (Rehmannia glutinosa)
- 9 grams of **Shan Zhu Yu** (Cornus)
- 9 grams of **Shan Yao** (Dioscorea)
- 9 grams of **Fu Ling** (Poria)
- 9 grams of **Mu Dan Pi** (Paeonia suffruticosa)
- 9 grams of **Ze Xie** (Water plantain)

Instructions Combine the ingredients in a pot with 500 mL of water. Bring to a boil, then simmer for 20-30 minutes. Strain and drink the decoction.

Application Liu Wei Di Huang Wan is used to nourish kidney Yin and regulate hormonal balance. It can treat symptoms such as irregular menstruation, night sweats, and hot flashes by supporting the kidney system.

Buplerum Peony Combination (Jia Wei Xiao Yao San)

Ingredients

- 9 grams of **Bai Shao** (Paeonia lactiflora)
- 9 grams of **Dang Gui** (Angelica sinensis)
- 9 grams **of Chuan Xiong** (Ligusticum chuanxiong)
- 12 grams of **Bai Zhu** (Atractylodes macrocephala)
- 12 grams of **Fu Ling** (Poria)
- 6 grams of **Gan Cao** (Licorice)
- 9 grams of **Bo He** (Peppermint)
- 12 grams of **Mu Dan Pi** (Paeonia suffruticosa)
- 9 grams of **Zhi Zi** (Gardenia)

Instructions Combine the ingredients in a pot with 500 mL of water. Bring to a boil, then simmer for 20-30 minutes. Strain and drink the decoction.

Application Jia Wei Xiao Yao San is used to treat PMS, irritability, and irregular menstruation. It regulates Liver Qi, tonifies Spleen Qi, and nourishes the blood, promoting emotional and physical balance.

Four Substance Decoction with Peach Pit (Tao Hong Si Wu Tang)

Ingredients

- 9 grams of **Dang Gui** (Angelica sinensis)
- 9 grams of **Chuan Xiong** (Ligusticum chuanxiong)
- 12 grams of **Bai Shao** (Paeonia lactiflora)
- 12 grams of **Shu Di Huang** (Rehmannia glutinosa)
- 9 grams of **Tao Ren** (Peach kernel)
- 89 grams of **Hong Hua** (Safflower)

Instructions Combine the ingredients in a pot with 500 mL of water. Bring to a boil, then simmer for 20-30 minutes. Strain and drink the decoction.

Application Tao Hong Si Wu Tang is used to treat irregular menstruation, blood stasis, and painful periods. It invigorates blood circulation and dispels stasis.

Tiao Yuan Duo Zi Fang (Rehmannia and Multi-seed Decoction)

Ingredients

- 9 grams of **Shu Di Huang** (Rehmannia glutinosa)
- 9 grams of **Dang Gui** (Angelica sinensis)
- 9 grams of **Bai Shao** (Paeonia lactiflora)
- 9 grams of **Shan Yao** (Dioscorea opposita)

- 6 grams of **Gan Cao** (Licorice)
- 9 grams of **Tu Si Zi** (Cuscuta chinensis)
- 9 grams of **Sha Ren** (Amomum)
- 9 grams of **Lu Jiao** (Deer antler glue) or a suitable substitute, such as **Shan Zhu Yu** (Cornus officinalis)
- 9 grams of **Rou Cong Rong** (Cistanche deserticola)
- 6 grams of **Wu Wei Zi** (Schisandra chinensis)

Instructions Combine the ingredients in a pot with 500 mL of water. Bring to a boil, then simmer for 20-30 minutes. Strain and drink the decoction.

Application Tiao Yuan Duo Zi Fang is a formula that is commonly used to improve fertility and support reproductive health in women. It nourishes Kidney essence (Jing) and Qi, which are essential for reproductive function. By strengthening the Kidney, this formula promotes hormonal balance and supports the production of healthy eggs. Additionally, it can also help with other symptoms of reproductive health issues such as fatigue and cold extremities. Always consult a qualified TCM practitioner before beginning any new herbal treatment.

Dang Gui Shao Yao San (Dang Gui and Peony Powder)

Ingredients

- 9 grams of **Dang Gui** (Angelica sinensis)
- 9 grams of **Bai Shao** (Paeonia lactiflora)
- 12 grams of **Chuan Xiong** (Ligusticum chuanxiong)
- 9 grams of **Bai Zhu** (Atractylodes macrocephala)
- 9 grams of **Fu Ling** (Poria)
- 9 grams of **Ze Xie** (Water plantain)

Instructions Combine the ingredients in a pot with 500 mL of water. Bring to a boil, then simmer for 20-30 minutes. Strain and drink the decoction.

Application Dang Gui Shao Yao San is used to treat symptoms such as irregular periods and water retention. It supports Liver and Spleen function, regulates Qi and Blood, and reduces dampness.

If you would like to make a bigger batch ahead, you can do so by increasing the amount of ingredients proportionally to the amount of water. Keep the decoction simmering for 5 minutes longer for every additional 100ml of water plus the proportionally increased amount of herbs. When you are consuming the ready-made batch, make sure to keep the decoction warm for consumption.

Remember, these formulations are just general guidelines, and the actual prescription may vary based on an individual's unique constitution and health needs. Always consult with a qualified TCM practitioner before using any herbal remedies.

Integrating Herbal Remedies into Daily Life

While these herbal remedies offer powerful support for menstrual health, their effectiveness is enhanced when combined with mindful lifestyle practices. TCM emphasizes the importance of balanced nutrition, stress management, and harmonizing daily routines to complement the use of herbs. As with any form of medicine, it is advised to consult with a qualified TCM practitioner to tailor herbal formulations to individual needs and for ensuring optimal results.

In the chapters ahead, a variety of themes such as specific TCM practices, dietary recommendations, and lifestyle adjustments that synergize with herbal remedies will be introduced to offer a holistic approach to restore feminine reproductive health. As we explore the world of herbal interventions in TCM, let us embrace the richness of nature's pharmacy and unlock the potential for profound healing in women's reproductive health.

6

TCM Modalities for Menstrual Irregularities

In this chapter, we delve into TCM modalities, specifically tailored to address menstrual irregularities and associated ailments. Through centuries of observation and practice, TCM offers holistic approaches to promote balance and harmony within the body, restoring menstrual health and vitality. Here are some of the key TCM modalities, including acupuncture and vaginal steam, and how they can effectively alleviate discomfort and diseases related to menstrual irregularities.

Acupuncture

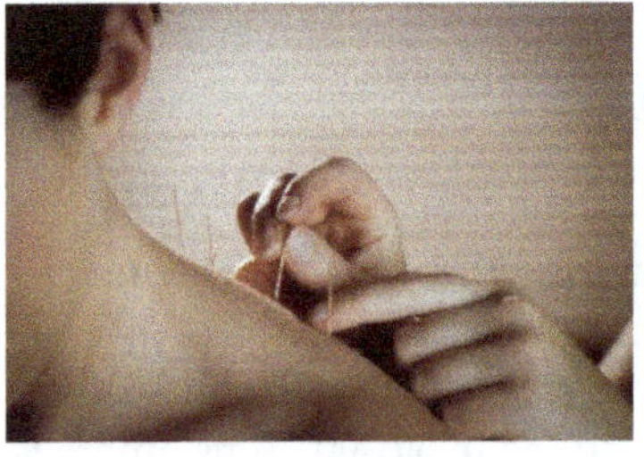

Acupuncture is a healing practice that originated in China over 2,000 years ago and is a central part of Traditional Chinese Medicine (TCM). It involves inserting very thin needles into specific points on the body to stimulate the flow of Qi (pronounced "chee"), or vital energy. Qi flows through pathways called **meridians,** and when the flow of Qi is disrupted, it can lead to health problems. By inserting needles into specific points along these meridians, acupuncture can restore the balance of Qi and promote overall health and well-being.

The history of acupuncture is deeply rooted in ancient Chinese medical texts, such as the *Huangdi Neijing* (The Yellow Emperor's Classic of Medicine), one of the oldest and most comprehensive TCM texts. This text outlines the theory of meridians and acupoints, describing how they connect different parts of the body and influence various organs and functions. Classical texts like the *Huangdi Neijing* form the foundation of TCM and provide insights into the practice and theory of acupuncture.

Acupuncture is known for its ability to treat a wide range of health conditions, including hormonal imbalances. Numerous published studies have demonstrated the efficacy of acupuncture for this purpose. For example, a study by Manheimer, E., et al., published in 2017 and titled "Effects of Acupuncture on Fertility Outcomes in Women With PCOS Undergoing in vitro fertilization Treatment: A Randomized Controlled Trial" demonstrated how acupuncture can enhance the success of in vitro fertilization in women with polycystic ovarian syndrome (PCOS).

In modern-day China and other East Asian countries, acupuncture is widely accepted and integrated into the healthcare system. It is recognized as an effective treatment for various conditions and is often used alongside conventional medical treatments. Patients in these countries have access to both traditional and modern medical practices, including acupuncture.

The process is generally safe and minimally invasive, and most people find it to be a relaxing and therapeutic experience. If you have any concerns or specific health issues, always consult with your healthcare provider before trying acupuncture

Vaginal Steam

Vaginal steam, also known as yoni steam, is a traditional practice rooted in TCM and other indigenous healing traditions. This gentle therapy involves sitting over a steaming herbal infusion, allowing the medicinal properties of the herbs to permeate the vaginal tissues and pelvic region. Vaginal steam supports circulation, reduces inflammation, and nurtures the reproductive organs.

Vaginal steam is believed to regulate Qi and blood flow in the pelvic region, addressing stagnation and resolving dampness and cold that may contribute to menstrual irregularities. The warmth and moisture of the steam also nourish Yin energy, promoting hormonal balance and alleviating discomfort.

Traditional Chinese medicine includes the practice of herbal baths for promoting health and recovery, particularly for postpartum women. These methods often involve infusing herbs in hot water and allowing the body to absorb the steam and heat. Vaginal steaming may have evolved from these practices as a targeted approach to addressing reproductive health issues.

In classical TCM texts, there are references to the use of steam therapy and herbal remedies for women's health, particularly in the treatment of gynecological issues.

A notable text is *Jia Yi Jing* (The Fine Art of Pregnancy and Childbirth), which discusses Chinese obstetrics and gynecology. It includes references to vaginal steaming and its effects on promoting postpartum recovery, regulating menstruation, and alleviating gynecological conditions.

According to historical TCM texts, regular vaginal steaming can help improve following symptoms:

Menstrual Irregularities

Vaginal steaming may help regulate menstrual cycles and alleviate symptoms such as heavy bleeding, spotting, or irregular periods.

Menstrual Cramps

The warmth and herbal steam may help soothe and reduce menstrual pain and cramping.

Dryness

Steam can add moisture to the vaginal area and may help relieve dryness.

Infections

Some believe that steaming with specific herbs can help reduce the risk of yeast infections and bacterial vaginosis.

Postpartum Healing

Vaginal steaming may be used to support postpartum recovery by promoting circulation and healing in the vaginal area.

Stress and Relaxation

The process can be calming and may help reduce stress and promote relaxation.

Digestive Issues

Vaginal steaming can improve circulation in the lower abdomen, potentially aiding digestion.

Hemorrhoids

The warmth and steam may provide relief from hemorrhoids in the perineal area, which in time can relieve itchiness and reduce the size of the hemorrhoids.

How to Perform Vaginal Steam at Home

Ingredients
✓   2-3 tablespoons of dried herbs
✓   2-4 cups of boiling water

❖ Tools Needed

Steaming Vessel

A pot or basin where you will place the herbs and hot water to create the steam. Choose a size that fits your needs and the space where you plan to steam.

Heat Source

A stove or other means to heat water to the appropriate temperature. Avoid boiling the water vigorously to minimize the risk of scalding. Electric countertop stove with adjustable heat is recommended.

Seat or Stool

A seat with an open base or a special vaginal steam chair that allows you to sit comfortably over the steaming vessel. Ensure it is stable and comfortable. A portable toilet (for camping) is perfect for this purpose.

Towels or Blankets

Towels or blankets can be used to create a tent-like structure around the seat and steaming vessel to trap the steam and keep you warm during the session.

Timer

Use a timer to keep track of the steaming session and avoid staying in the steam for too long.

❖ Commonly Used TCM Herbs for Vaginal Steam

Mugwort Ai Ye, *Artemisia argyi*
 Mugwort is a key herb in TCM known for its ability to warm the uterus, regulate menstrual cycles, and alleviate menstrual cramps. It is believed to promote circulation and dispel cold from the pelvic region.

Motherwort Yi Mu Cao, *Leonurus japonicus*
Motherwort is valued in TCM for its ability to regulate menstruation, alleviate menstrual pain, and support overall reproductive health. It is thought to invigorate Qi and blood flow in the uterus.

Dang Gui *Angelica sinensis*
Also known as "female ginseng," Dang Gui is a revered herb in TCM for women's health. It is commonly used to tonify blood, regulate menstrual cycles, and alleviate symptoms of menstrual irregularities such as amenorrhea and dysmenorrhea.

Tangerine Peel Ju Pi, *Citrus Reticulata*
Tangerine peel is a frequently used herb in TCM formulas that regulates Qi and relieves bloating while promoting healthy digestion and facilitating absorption of nutrients. It can help balance hormonal fluctuations.

Red Sage Dan Shen, *Salvia miltiorrhiza*
Red sage is a commonly used herb in TCM that supports overall reproductive health. It reduces inflammation and supports the healing process by promoting blood circulation and accelerating the breakdown of blood stasis.

Calendula *Calendula officinalis*
Calendula has anti-inflammatory and antispasmodic properties and is often included in vaginal steam blends to soothe pelvic discomfort, promote tissue healing, and support overall reproductive health.

Nutgrass Xiang Fu, Cyperus rotundus
Xiang Fu is one of the key herbs in TCM that has neutral temperature characteristic. It regulates menstruation and alleviates menstrual pain by soothing the Liver and relieving emotional stress. Helps balance hormones and improve mood.

Dandelion Leaves Pu Gong Ying Ye, Taraxacum officinale
Dandelion leaves are known to have a cooling nature in TCM. Its anti-inflammatory properties can help soothe irritation and reduce inflammation while balancing moisture level to maintain a healthy environment in the vaginal area.

❖ Instructions:

1. Place the dried herbs in a large heatproof bowl or pot.

2. Carefully pour the boiling water over the herbs, covering them completely.

3. Allow the herbal infusion to steep for 5-10 minutes, then place the bowl or pot in a comfortable and safe location.

4. Sit over the steam, ensuring a safe distance to avoid burns, and cover yourself with a blanket or towel to retain the heat.

5. Relax and enjoy the steam for 15-30 minutes, allowing the medicinal properties of the herbs to penetrate the pelvic region.

6. After the steam session, rest for a few minutes and avoid exposure to cold drafts.

While some of these herbs may not be as readily available in North America and Europe, they can often be found in specialized health food stores, herbal apothecaries, or online retailers that specialize in TCM herbs and remedies. It's important to source high-quality herbs from reputable suppliers to ensure their safety and efficacy.

❖ Additional Considerations

- Consult with a healthcare professional before trying vaginal steam, especially if you have any pre-existing health conditions or concerns.

- Use caution when handling hot water or steam to avoid burns or scalds.

- Discontinue vaginal steam if you experience any pain, discomfort, or adverse reactions. Seek medical attention if necessary in such case.

- Do not attempt vaginal steam during menstruation or if you are pregnant. It may pose risks to your health if you attempt during those times.

- Ensure proper hygiene and sanitation of equipment and surroundings to minimize the risk of infection.

- Stay hydrated and listen to your body's cues during vaginal steam sessions, taking breaks as needed.

Moxibustion

Moxibustion is a traditional Chinese medicine therapy that involves the burning of dried mugwort (Artemisia argyi) on or near the skin to stimulate specific acupuncture points and meridians. For thousands of years, it has been utilized to promote health.Moxibustion works by stimulating the flow of Qi and blood along meridians (energy pathways) in the body. This helps to balance the body's internal energies and promote overall

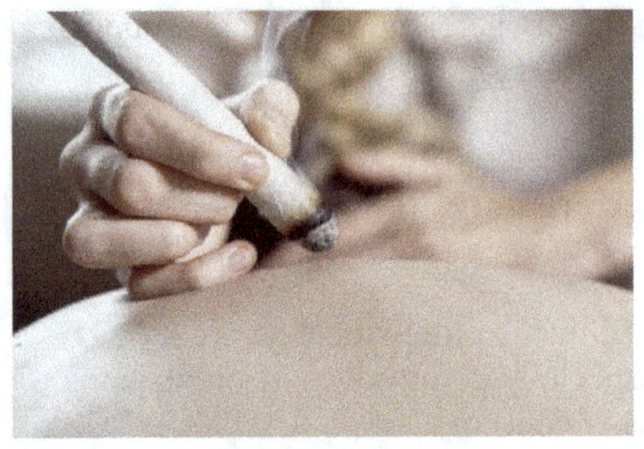

health. The burning mugwort creates a warming effect on the area where it is applied, which helps to promote the flow of Qi and blood, especially in areas where there may be stagnation or blockages. Moxibustion is often applied to specific acupoints that are associated with different organs or functions in the body, enhancing their natural functions.

By warming areas that may be too cold or deficient, it clears cold and dampness, which can cause stagnation and pain, particularly in the lower abdomen and reproductive organs. The therapy also supports digestive health by promoting the smooth flow of Qi and blood in the abdomen. In regard to women's health, moxibustion can help regulate the menstrual cycle and relieve menstrual pain by improving circulation and energy flow in the reproductive organs. Always consult a qualified TCM practitioner for guidance before trying moxibustion, as they can provide personalized advice and treatment plans.

While moxibustion can be performed at home, it is highly recommended to seek guidance from a qualified practitioner to ensure safe and effective application. Practitioners can provide personalized advice on which points to stimulate and the appropriate amount of heat.To apply moxibustion to oneself, you will need a few specific tools and supplies. It is essential to follow safety precautions and seek guidance from a qualified Traditional Chinese Medicine (TCM) practitioner before attempting self-treatment.

❖ **Tools and Supplies Needed:**

✓ **Mugwort** The primary herb used for moxibustion is dried mugwort (Artemisia argyi). It can be found in various forms such as moxa sticks, moxa cones, or loose moxa wool.

✓ **Moxa Sticks** These are cylindrical sticks made of compressed mugwort. They are often used for indirect moxibustion and can be lit and held close to the skin.

Or **Moxa Cones** Small cones of mugwort that can be burned directly on the skin or on a barrier (such as a slice of ginger, garlic, or salt) placed on the skin.

✓ **Barrier Materials** For indirect moxibustion, materials such as ginger, garlic, salt, or a thin slice of another protective barrier may be used to place between the moxa cone and the skin.

✓ **Lighter or Matches** To ignite the moxa stick or cone.

✓ **Tweezers** Helpful for handling the moxa cones and adjusting their placement.

✓ **Heat-Resistant Surface** A surface to safely extinguish and store the moxa stick or cone when not in use.

✓ **Alcohol and Cotton Swabs** Useful for cleaning the skin and moxa tools as needed.

❖ How Moxibustion is Applied:

Preparation:

- Select the appropriate form of moxibustion (moxa stick or moxa cone) based on the treatment and area to be stimulated.

- Choose the acupuncture points you wish to treat.

- Ensure the skin is clean and dry before beginning.

Application:

- For indirect moxibustion, place a barrier (such as a slice of ginger or garlic) on the selected acupuncture point.

- Light the moxa stick or cone using a lighter or matches.

- Hold the lit moxa stick about 1-2 inches away from the skin over the chosen acupuncture point or place the lit moxa cone on the barrier over the point.

- Move the moxa stick in small circles or hold it in place until you feel a comfortable warming sensation.

Safety and Monitoring

- Be careful not to let the moxa burn too close to the skin to avoid burns.

- Monitor the temperature and move the moxa stick or cone away if it becomes too hot.

- Treatments typically last a few minutes per point or as recommended by a practitioner.

Finishing

- Extinguish the moxa stick or cone safely on a heat-resistant surface.

- Clean the area if necessary and store your tools properly.

❖ Where to Apply Moxibustion

While many acupoints on the body can contribute to reproductive health, certain points on the hand and the sole of the foot are particularly important for promoting balance and energy flow in the reproductive system. Here are six meridian points on the hand and the sole where moxibustion can be applied:

Pericardium 6 (Nèiguān, PC 6)

- Located about three finger widths above the wrist crease on the inner side of the forearm.
- Stimulating this point can help regulate hormones and ease emotional stress, which are important for reproductive health.

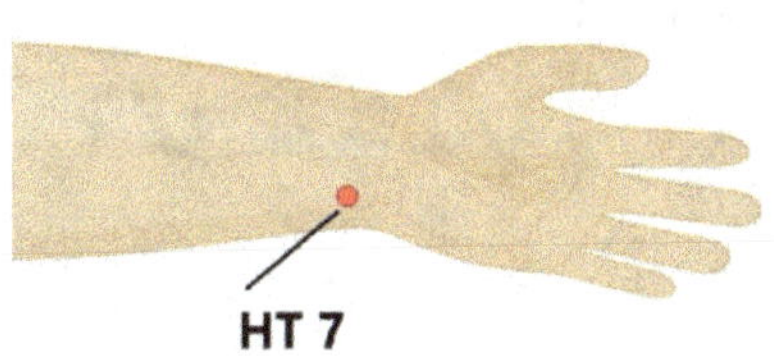

Heart 7 (Shénmén, HT 7)

- Located at the base of the wrist on the inner side of the arm, in line with the pinky finger.
- Moxibustion on this point can help balance emotions, promote calmness, and support overall well-being.

Lung 9 (Tàiyuān, LU 9)

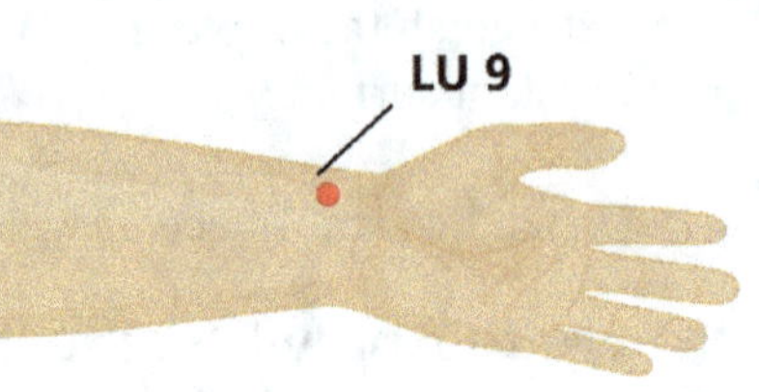

- Located at the wrist crease on the inner side of the thumb.
- Stimulating this point can help improve blood circulation and support healthy breathing, which is important for overall health and vitality.

Kidney 1 (Yǒngquán, KD 1)

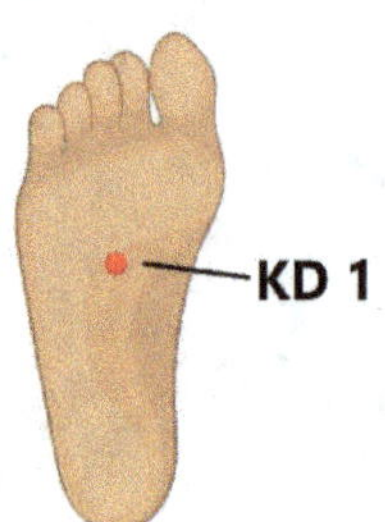

- Located on the sole of the foot, about one-third of the way down from the base of the toes.
- Known as the "Gushing Spring," this point is believed to help ground the body and support overall energy flow.

Spleen 1 (Yǐnbái, SP 1)

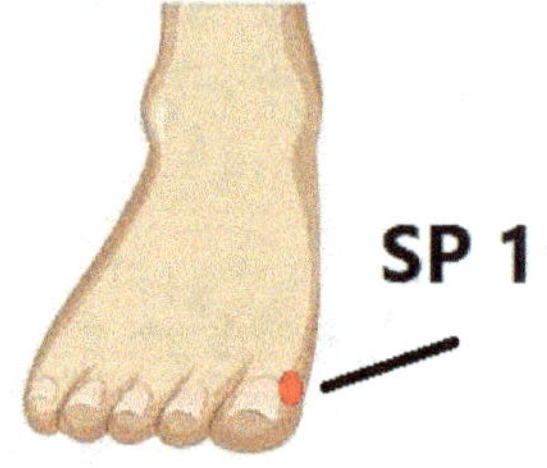

- Located on the medial side of the big toe, just at the nail's edge.
- Stimulating this point can help support menstrual health and regulate the cycle.

Bladder 60 (Kūnlún,Wis BD 60)

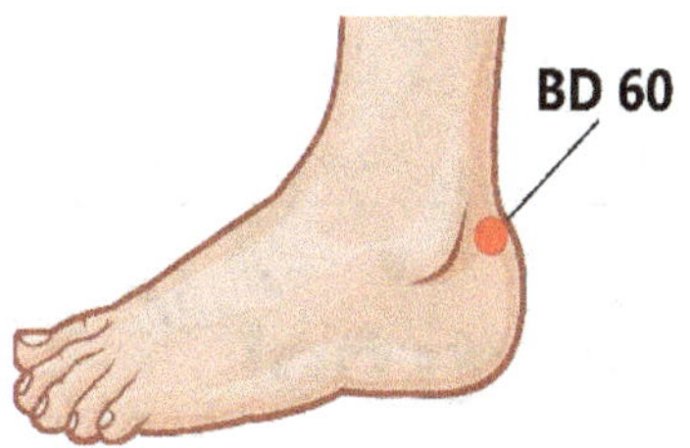

-     Located at the midpoint between the lateral malleolus (outer ankle bone) and the Achilles tendon on the back of the foot.
-     Moxibustion on this point can promote smooth blood circulation and support the lower back and reproductive organs.

These meridian points play a significant role in promoting fertility and regulating menstrual cycles according to TCM principles. By using moxibustion on these points, one can aim to improve energy flow, balance hormones, and support overall reproductive health. Always seek guidance from a qualified TCM practitioner to ensure proper technique and safety during moxibustion treatments.

❖ Additional Considerations:

- **Safety**: Always prioritize safety and avoid using moxibustion if you have certain conditions (e.g., skin sensitivity, open wounds).

- Seek guidance from a licensed practitioner for proper application and treatment duration.

- Perform moxibustion in a well-ventilated area to avoid excessive smoke inhalation.

7

Nutrition for Menstrual Wellness in Traditional Chinese Medicine

In Traditional Chinese Medicine (TCM), nutrition is viewed as a powerful tool for maintaining balance and promoting optimal health. The foods we consume are believed to have specific energetic properties that influence the body's internal balance of Yin and Yang, as well as the flow of Qi and blood. This chapter explores key nutritional principles rooted in TCM that support menstrual wellness and hormonal balance.

Harmonizing Yin and Yang: Balancing Opposing Forces

TCM categorizes foods based on their inherent energetic qualities, with Yin and Yang representing opposing yet complementary forces. Balancing the consumption of Yin and Yang foods is essential for harmonizing the menstrual cycle and supporting overall health.

Yin Foods

Cool and moist in nature, Yin foods nourish and moisturize the body, promoting relaxation and fluidity. Examples include leafy greens, cucumbers, watermelon, tofu, and seaweed. Incorporating Yin foods during menstruation and the follicular phase can help replenish fluids and cool excess heat.

Examples of Yin Foods: leafy greens, cucumbers, watermelon, tofu, seaweed, fruits

Yang Foods

Warm and drying in nature, Yang foods invigorate and energize the body, promoting warmth and activity. Examples include ginger, garlic, cinnamon, lamb, and chicken. Consuming Yang foods during the ovulatory and luteal phases can support energy levels and vitality.

Examples of Yang Foods: ginger, garlic, spices, cinnamon, spicy peppers, lamb, chicken

Nourishing Blood and Qi: Supporting Vital Energies

Adequate nourishment of blood and Qi is crucial for menstrual health and overall well-being in TCM. Certain foods are prized for their ability to tonify blood and Qi, promoting vitality and regulating the menstrual cycle.

Blood-Tonifying Foods

Foods rich in iron, vitamin C, and B vitamins are beneficial for nourishing blood. Examples include dark leafy greens, beets, blackstrap molasses, dates, and red meat. Incorporating these foods throughout the menstrual cycle can help prevent blood deficiency and alleviate symptoms of anemia.

Qi-Tonifying Foods

Foods that strengthen Qi and promote circulation are essential for sustaining energy levels and vitality. Examples include whole

grains, legumes, nuts, seeds, and warming spices like ginger and
cinnamon. Including Qi-tonifying foods in the diet supports
overall resilience and hormonal balance.

Clearing Heat and Dampness: Alleviating Excess

Excess heat and dampness in the body can disrupt the menstrual
cycle and lead to symptoms such as heavy periods, bloating, and
inflammation. Choosing foods with cooling and drying
properties can help clear heat and dampness, restoring balance.

Cooling Foods

Foods with cooling properties help clear heat and reduce
inflammation in the body. Examples include cucumber, celery,
mung beans, watermelon, and bitter greens like dandelion and
kale. Consuming cooling foods during the menstrual phase and
in hot weather can help alleviate heat-related symptoms.

Drying Foods

Foods with drying properties help resolve dampness and promote
fluid balance in the body. Examples include barley, adzuki
beans, radish, and bitter melon. Incorporating drying foods
during the luteal phase can help reduce bloating and water
retention.

Moderating Spicy and Stimulating Foods: Regulating Energy Flow

While spices and stimulants can invigorate circulation and
digestion, excessive consumption may disrupt the body's internal
balance and exacerbate symptoms of heat and Qi stagnation.
Moderation is key when incorporating these foods into the diet.

Moderating Spices

Spices such as chili peppers, cayenne, and black pepper have warming properties that can promote circulation but may aggravate heat-related symptoms if consumed excessively. Use spices mindfully and in moderation, especially during the menstrual phase.

Limiting Stimulants

Stimulants like caffeine and alcohol can overstimulate the body's systems, leading to Qi stagnation and Yin deficiency over time. Limiting intake of caffeinated beverages and alcoholic drinks can support hormonal balance and reduce stress on the body.

Hydration and Fluid Balance: Nourishing Yin

Adequate hydration is essential for nourishing Yin and supporting fluid balance in the body, particularly during menstruation when blood and fluids are lost. Choosing hydrating foods and beverages can help replenish fluids and prevent dehydration.

Hydrating Foods

Foods with high water content, such as fruits and vegetables, contribute to hydration and promote fluid balance. Examples include watermelon, cucumber, oranges, and tomatoes. Consuming hydrating foods throughout the menstrual cycle supports Yin nourishment and overall hydration.

Herbal Teas

Herbal teas made from cooling and nourishing herbs, such as chrysanthemum, mint, and hibiscus, can help cool excess heat and replenish fluids. Enjoying herbal teas as part of a balanced diet promotes hydration and supports menstrual wellness.

Recipes for Harmonizing Qi, Building Blood and Nourishing the Body

Incorporating TCM-inspired recipes into your diet offers a delicious and effective way to support health and promote overall well-being. These recipes are thoughtfully crafted to harness the energetic properties of ingredients and align with TCM principles to nourish the body, regulate the menstrual cycle, and harmonize Qi flow.

Nourishing Blood Beet Salad (Vegetarian)

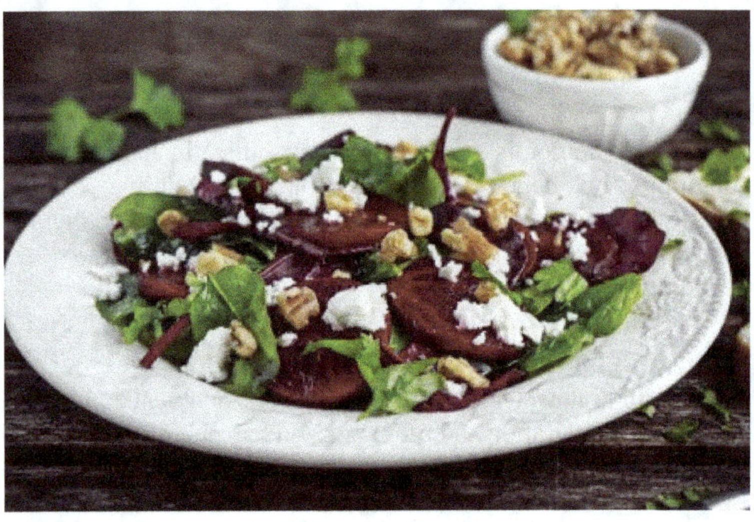

This vibrant salad is rich in iron, vitamin C, and B vitamins, essential nutrients for nourishing blood and supporting menstrual health. Beets, known for their blood-tonifying properties in TCM, are combined with leafy greens and seeds to create a nourishing dish that promotes vitality and resilience. Beets have a cooling and sweet nature that nourishes the blood and clears heat from the body. Leafy greens such as spinach and arugula are cooling in nature and support Liver.

function, promoting smooth Qi flow and reducing stagnation.

Ingredients:

- 2 medium beets roasted and sliced
- 2 cups baby spinach
- 1 cup arugula
- ¼ cup chopped walnuts
- (optional) ½ cup crumbled feta cheese
- Dressing: 2 tablespoons olive oil, 1 tablespoon balsamic vinegar, 1 teaspoon honey, salt, and pepper to taste

Instructions:

1. Preheat the oven to 400°F (200°C). Wrap the beets individually in foil and roast for 45-60 minutes, until tender. Let cool, then peel and slice.
2. In a large bowl, combine the roasted beets, baby spinach, arugula, pumpkin seeds, and feta cheese (if using).
3. In a small bowl, whisk together the olive oil, balsamic vinegar, honey, salt, and pepper to make the dressing.
4. Pour the dressing over the salad and gently toss to mix.

Qi-Boosting Ginger Chicken Stir-Fry

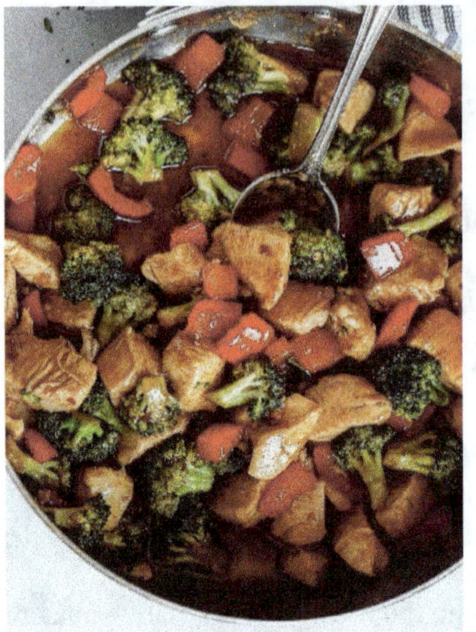

This savory stir-fry combines lean chicken breast with warming spices like ginger and garlic to invigorate Qi flow and support energy levels. Bell peppers and broccoli add color and crunch while providing essential nutrients for overall well-being.

Ginger and garlic are prized in TCM for their ability to warm the body, promote circulation, and dispel cold. Chicken is considered a Qi-tonifying food that nourishes the Spleen and Stomach, supporting digestion and energy production.

Ingredients:

- 1 lb (450g) boneless, skinless chicken breast, diced
- 1 tablespoon sesame oil
- 2 cloves garlic, minced
- 1 tablespoon fresh ginger, grated
- 1 red bell pepper, diced
- 1 cup broccoli florets
- 2 tablespoons soy sauce or tamari
- 1 tablespoon rice vinegar
- 1 teaspoon honey
- Cooked brown rice or quinoa, to serve with

Instructions:

1. Heat the sesame oil in a large skillet or wok over medium-high heat. Add the garlic and ginger, and sauté for 1-2 minutes until fragrant.
2. Add the diced chicken breast to the skillet and stir-fry until cooked through, about 5-6 minutes.
3. Add the cut bell pepper and broccoli florets to the skillet, and stir-fry for an additional 3-4 minutes until tender-crisp.
4. In a small bowl, whisk together the soy sauce, rice vinegar, and honey. Pour the sauce over the chicken and vegetables and toss to coat evenly.
5. Serve the stir-fry hot over cooked brown rice or quinoa, garnished with chopped green onions or sesame seeds if desired.

Cooling Cucumber-Mint Smoothie (Vegetarian)

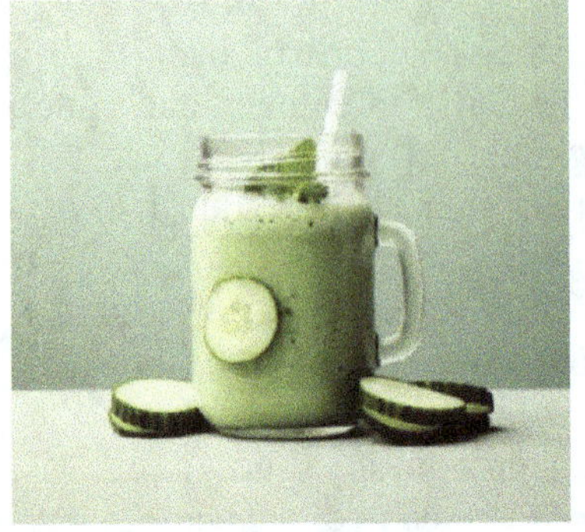

This refreshing smoothie combines hydrating cucumber with cooling mint and yogurt to soothe heat and promote fluid balance in the body. Rich in antioxidants and vitamins, this smoothie is a delicious way to support menstrual wellness and overall hydration.

Cucumber and mint are cooling in nature and help clear heat and dampness from the body, making them ideal for relieving heat-related symptoms during menstruation. Yogurt nourishes the Spleen and Stomach, supporting digestion and harmonizing Qi flow. Although this is a 'cooling' recipe, try not to drink it too cold to help the digestive system function optimally.

Ingredients:

- 1 cucumber, peeled and chopped
- ½ cup fresh mint leaves
- 1 cup plain Greek yogurt
- 1 tablespoon honey (optional)
- ½ cup water or coconut water

Instructions:

1. In a blender, combine the chopped cucumber, fresh mint leaves, Greek yogurt, honey (if using), and water or coconut water.
2. Blend on high speed until smooth consistency, adding extra water as necessary to get the desired consistency.
3. Pour the smoothie into glasses and serve immediately, garnished with a sprig of fresh mint for a refreshing and nourishing treat.

Warming Lentil Soup with Turmeric and Spinach

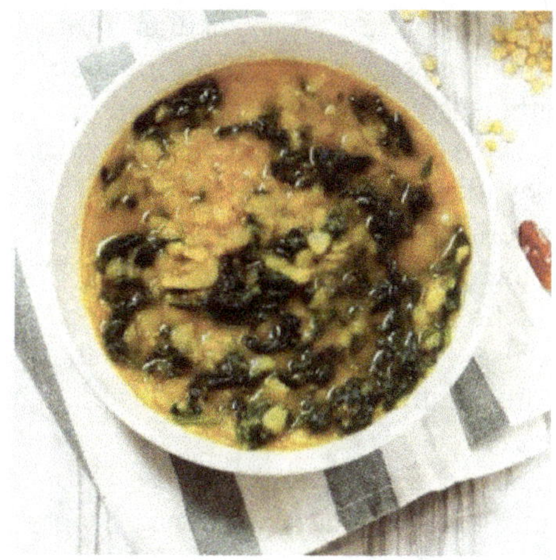

(Vegan)

This hearty lentil soup combines warming spices like turmeric and ginger with protein-rich lentils and nutrient-packed spinach. Perfect for colder days, this soup promotes circulation, supports digestion, and provides essential nutrients for menstrual wellness.

Ingredients:

- 1 cup dried brown lentils, rinsed and drained
- 1 onion, chopped
- 3 cloves garlic, minced
- 1 tablespoon fresh ginger, grated
- 1 teaspoon ground turmeric
- 1 teaspoon ground cumin
- ½ teaspoon ground coriander
- 4 cups vegetable broth
- 2 cups water
- 2 cups baby spinach leaves
- Salt and pepper to taste
- Fresh cilantro leaves for garnish (optional)

Instructions:

1. In a large pot, heat a bit of olive oil over medium heat. Add the chopped onion and stir fry on a pan for about 5 minutes, or until softened.
2. Stir in the minced garlic and grated ginger, and cook for another 1-2 minutes until fragrant.
3. Add the ground turmeric, cumin, and coriander to the pot, and stir to coat the onions and spices.
4. Pour in the vegetable broth and water, then add the rinsed lentils. Bring the soup to a boil, then reduce the heat to low, cover, and simmer for 20-25 minutes until the lentils are tender.
5. Stir in the baby spinach leaves and cook for an additional 2-3 minutes until wilted. Add salt and pepper to taste.
6. Ladle the soup into bowls and garnish with fresh cilantro leaves if desired. Serve hot and enjoy this nourishing and comforting dish!

Ginger-Turmeric Baked Salmon with Roasted Vegetables

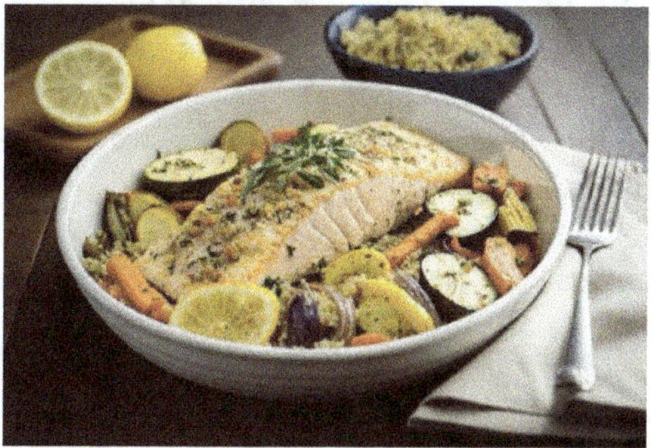

This flavorful and aromatic dish features omega-3 rich salmon fillets marinated in a warming blend of ginger, turmeric, and garlic. Paired with colorful roasted vegetables, this meal provides essential nutrients, supports circulation, and nourishes the body during the menstrual cycle.

Ingredients:

- 4 salmon fillets
- 2 tablespoons olive oil
- 1 tablespoon fresh ginger, grated
- 1 tablespoon fresh turmeric, grated (or 1 teaspoon ground turmeric)
- 2 cloves garlic, minced
- Zest and juice of 1 lemon
- Salt and pepper to taste
- 4 cups mixed vegetables (such as bell peppers, zucchini, cherry tomatoes, and red onion), chopped
- Fresh herb sprigs for garnish

Instructions:

1. Preheat the oven to 400°F (200°C). Use parchment paper to line a baking sheet.

2. In a small bowl, whisk together the olive oil, grated ginger, grated turmeric, minced garlic, lemon zest, and lemon juice to make the marinade.

3. Place the salmon fillets on the prepared baking sheet, and brush the marinade over the top of each fillet. Season with salt and pepper to taste.
4. Arrange the chopped mixed vegetables around the salmon on the baking sheet. Drizzle with a bit of olive oil and season with salt and pepper.
5. Bake for 12 to 15 minutes, or until the veggies are soft and the salmon is cooked through, in a preheated oven.
6. Take out of the oven, and before serving, top with fresh herb sprigs for garnish.

Warming Quinoa and Sweet Potato Buddha Bowl
(Vegan)

This nourishing Buddha bowl features quinoa, sweet potatoes, and warming spices like cinnamon and cumin. Rich in fiber, vitamins, and minerals, this hearty dish supports digestive health, stabilizes blood sugar levels, and provides essential nutrients for menstrual wellness.

Sweet potatoes and quinoa are considered neutral in nature and support Spleen and Stomach function, promoting digestion and nourishing Qi. Warming spices like cinnamon and cumin help invigorate Qi flow and dispel cold, supporting overall vitality and hormonal balance.

Ingredients:

- 1 cup quinoa, rinsed
- 2 cups water or vegetable broth
- 2 medium sweet potatoes, peeled and diced
- 1 tablespoon olive oil
- 1 teaspoon ground cinnamon
- 1 teaspoon ground cumin
- Salt and pepper to taste
- 2 cups mixed greens (such as spinach or kale)
- ½ cup chickpeas, drained and rinsed
- ¼ cup dried cranberries
- ¼ cup pumpkin seeds
- Tahini dressing or balsamic vinaigrette for serving

Instructions:

1. Preheat the oven to 400°F (200°C). Line a baking sheet with parchment paper.
2. Put water or vegetable broth with quinoa in a pan. Bring to a boil, then reduce the heat to low, cover, and simmer for 15-20 minutes until the quinoa is cooked and the liquid is absorbed.

3. While the quinoa is cooking, toss the diced sweet potatoes with olive oil, ground cinnamon, ground cumin, salt, and pepper on the prepared baking sheet. Roast in the preheated oven for 25-30 minutes until tender and lightly caramelized.
4. Divide the cooked quinoa, roasted sweet potatoes, mixed greens, chickpeas, dried cranberries, and pumpkin seeds among serving bowls.
5. Drizzle with tahini dressing or balsamic vinaigrette, and serve warm. Enjoy this nourishing and satisfying Buddha bowl that supports menstrual wellness and overall vitality!

Spicy Black Bean and Vegetable Stir-Fry (Vegan)

This spicy stir-fry features black beans, colorful vegetables, and aromatic spices like chili powder and paprika. Packed with protein, fiber, and essential nutrients, this flavorful dish supports digestive health, promotes circulation, and provides sustained energy for menstrual wellness.

Black beans are neutral in nature and nourish both Yin and Yang, making them ideal for supporting overall vitality and hormonal balance. Spices like chili powder and paprika have warming properties that help dispel cold and invigorate Qi flow, promoting energy and resilience.

Ingredients:

- 1 tablespoon olive oil
- 1 onion, thinly sliced
- 2 cloves garlic, minced
- 1 bell pepper, thinly sliced
- 1 zucchini, thinly sliced
- 1 cup sliced mushrooms
- 1 can (15 oz) black beans, drained and rinsed
- 1 teaspoon chili powder
- 1 teaspoon paprika
- Salt and pepper to taste
- Fresh cilantro for garnish
- Cooked brown rice or quinoa for serving

Instructions:

1. Heat the olive oil in a large skillet or wok over medium-high heat. Add the minced garlic and onion, and sauté for two to three minutes, or until aromatic.
2. Add the sliced bell pepper, zucchini, and mushrooms to the skillet, and stir-fry for 5-6 minutes until tender-crisp.

3. Stir in the black beans, chili powder, paprika, salt, and pepper, and cook for an additional 2-3 minutes until heated through.
4. Serve the spicy black bean and vegetable stir-fry over cooked brown rice or quinoa, garnished with fresh cilantro. Enjoy this flavorful and nutritious dish that supports menstrual wellness and satisfies the taste buds!

Hearty Chicken and Vegetable Soup with Ginger

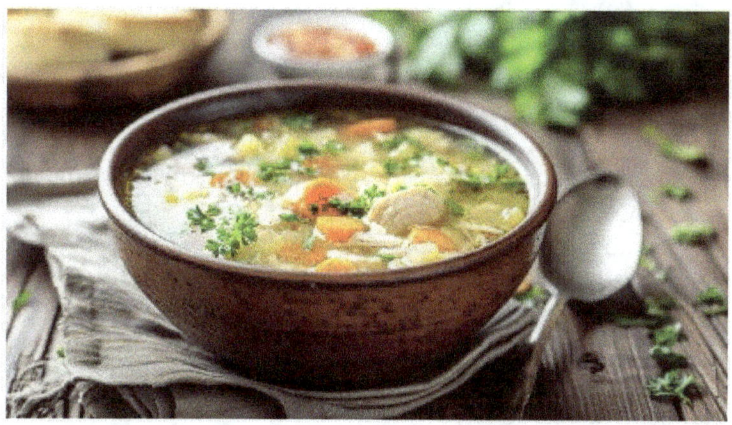

This comforting soup features tender chicken, nourishing vegetables, and warming ginger in a flavorful broth. Rich in protein, vitamins, and minerals, this wholesome dish supports immune function, promotes digestion, and provides essential nutrients that supports women's reproductive system.

Chicken is considered a Qi-tonifying food that nourishes the Spleen and Stomach, supporting digestion and energy production. Ginger is prized in TCM for its warming properties that promote circulation, dispel cold, and soothe digestive discomfort, making it ideal for supporting menstrual regulation.

Ingredients:

- 1 tablespoon olive oil
- 1 onion, chopped
- 3 cloves garlic, minced
- 1 tablespoon fresh ginger, grated
- 2 carrots, peeled and diced
- 2 celery stalks, diced
- 6 cups chicken broth
- 2 boneless, skinless chicken breasts, cut in bite size

- 1 cup chopped kale or spinach
- Salt and pepper to taste
- Fresh parsley for garnish

Instructions:

1. Heat the olive oil in a big pot over medium heat. Add the chopped onion, minced garlic, and grated ginger, and sauté for 2-3 minutes until fragrant.
2. Add the diced carrots and celery to the pot, and cook for another 3-4 minutes until slightly softened.
3. Add the chicken broth and bring to a boil. Add the diced chicken breasts to the pot, reduce the heat to low, cover, and simmer for 20-25 minutes until the chicken is cooked through.
4. Stir in the chopped kale or spinach and cook for an additional 2-3 minutes until wilted. Salt and pepper to taste.
5. Ladle the soup into a bowl, garnish with fresh parsley, and serve hot.

Nourishing Brown Rice Congee with Mushrooms and Spinach (Vegan)

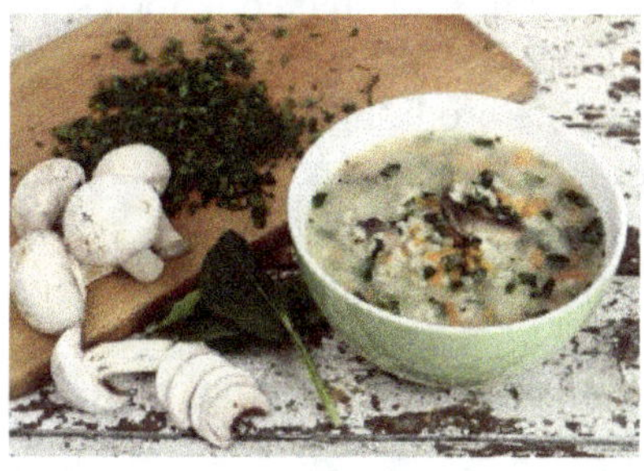

Congee, also known as rice porridge, is a staple in TCM for its gentle and nourishing properties. Brown rice is neutral in nature and supports the Spleen and Stomach, promoting digestion and nourishing Qi. Mushrooms are prized for their ability to tonify Qi and blood, while spinach adds a dose of cooling Yin energy to balance the dish.

Easy to digest and rich in vitamins and minerals, this savory dish supports digestive health, and nourishes Yin.

Ingredients:

- 1 cup brown rice
- 6 cups water or vegetable broth
- 1 tablespoon olive oil
- 1 onion, chopped
- 2 cloves garlic, minced
- 1 tablespoon fresh ginger, grated
- 1 cup mushrooms, sliced
- 2 cups baby spinach leaves
- 2 oz. carrots, grated (optional)
- Salt and pepper to taste
- Optional toppings: sliced green onions, toasted sesame seeds, tamari or soy sauce

Instructions:

1. Till the water runs clear, wash the brown rice under cold water. Drain and set aside.

2. Heat olive oil over medum heat in a big pot. Add the
    chopped onion, minced garlic, and grated ginger, and
    sauté for 2-3 minutes until fragrant.
3. Add the sliced mushrooms to the pot, and cook for
    another 4-5 minutes until tender.
4. Pour in the water or vegetable broth. Fill the pot with the
    washed brown rice. Bring to a boil, then reduce the heat
    to low, cover, and simmer for 45-60 minutes until the
    rice is soft and creamy, stirring occasionally.
5. Stir in the baby spinach leaves and cook for an
    additional 2-3 minutes until wilted. Season the congee
    with salt and pepper to taste.
6. Ladle the nourishing brown rice congee into bowls, and
    top with sliced green onions, toasted sesame seeds,
    grated carrots, and a drizzle of tamari or soy sauce if
    desired. Serve hot.

These TCM-inspired recipes offer flavorful and nutritious
options for promoting menstrual wellness and supporting overall
health. By incorporating these dishes into your diet along with
mindful eating practices, you can harness the healing power of
food to cultivate balance, vitality, and harmony in every phase of
the menstrual cycle.

8

Holistic Wellness According to TCM

The holistic approach in medicine recognizes the interconnectedness of the body, mind, and spirit, emphasizing comprehensive care that addresses underlying causes and promotes overall health and well-being. This chapter will present the integration of Traditional Chinese Medicine (TCM), physical movement, and mindfulness practices, recognizing the interconnectedness of body, mind, and spirit. By synergistically combining these modalities, you can cultivate a state of optimal health and well-being. Physical movement, including yoga, tai chi, and qigong, enhances circulation, flexibility, and strength while fostering a sense of embodiment and balance. Mindfulness practices, such as meditation and breathwork, cultivate present-moment awareness, reduce stress, and promote emotional resilience. You can benefit from these integrated practices by addressing menstrual irregularities, hormonal imbalances, and reproductive health concerns. By nurturing the body, calming the mind, and connecting with the inner self, you can experience profound benefits, including improved energy, mood, and overall quality of life.

Synergy between TCM and Physical Movement

Yoga

Yoga is an ancient practice that originated in India and focuses on physical postures, breath control, and meditation. From a TCM perspective, yoga promotes the smooth flow of Qi and balances the body's yin and yang. Certain yoga postures can help improve blood flow, reduce stress, and balance hormones. Here are some yoga postures that are beneficial for regulating menstrual cycles and promoting reproductive health, along with instructions on how to perform them.

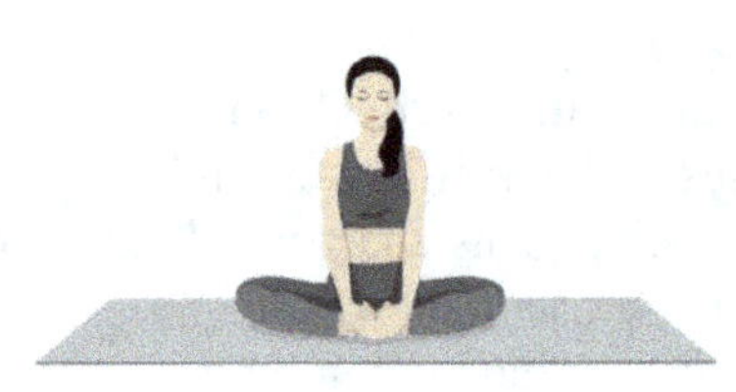

Baddha Konasana (Bound Angle Pose)

- Sit on the floor with your legs extended.
- Bring the soles of your feet together and bend your knees.
- Hold your feet with your hands and allow your knees to drop towards the floor.
- Keep your back straight and gently press your thighs down towards the ground.
- Breathe deeply while holding the pose for one to two minutes.

Supta Baddha Konasana (Reclining Bound Angle Pose)

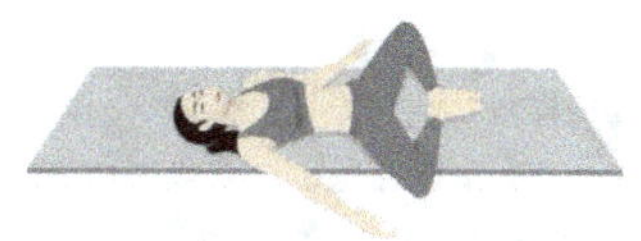

- Start in Baddha Konasana.
- Slowly lean back, supporting your upper body with your hands, and eventually lie down on the floor.
- Place a cushion or rolled-up towel under your head and back for comfort.
- Relax your arms at your sides.
- Hold the pose for one to two minutes while breathing deeply.

Viparita Karani (Legs-Up-The-Wall Pose)

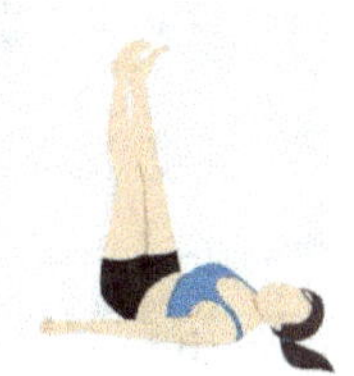

- Sit with one hip against a wall.
- Swing your legs up the wall as you lower your back onto the floor.
- Your buttocks should touch the wall, and your back should be flat on the ground.
- Rest your arms at your sides.
- Hold the pose for two to three minutes, focusing on deep, slow breathing.

Balasana (Child's Pose)

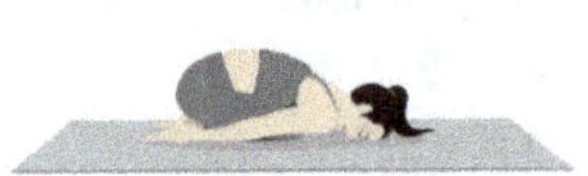

- Kneel on the floor with your big toes touching and knees slightly apart.
- Sit back on your heels and lower your forehead to the floor, extending your arms in front of you or resting them alongside your body.
- Relax your back and shoulders.
- Hold the pose for one to two minutes while breathing deeply.

Dandasana (Staff Pose)

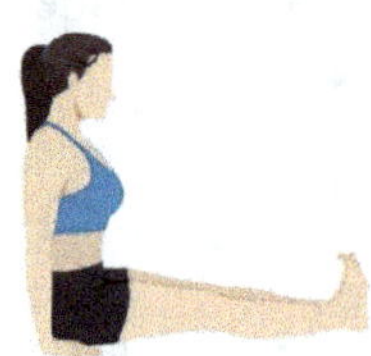

- Sit on the floor with your legs extended straight in front of you.
- Maintain a straight back and use your core.
- Place your hands on the floor beside your hips.
- Hold the pose for one minute while focusing on your breath.

Setu Bandhasana (Bridge Pose)

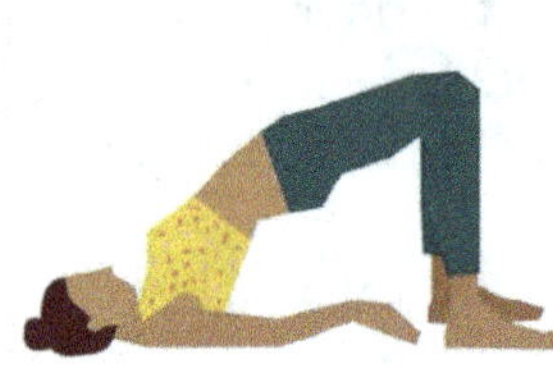

- Lie on your back with your knees bent. Keep your feet flat on the floor hip-width apart.
- Lift your hips towards the ceiling while pressing down on your arms and shoulders.
- Keep your back straight and avoid arching too much.
- Hold the pose for 30 seconds to 1 minute, then release and relax.

These yoga postures can help regulate menstrual cycles and support reproductive health by improving blood circulation to the pelvic area, reducing stress, and promoting relaxation.

Always listen to your body and modify poses as needed to ensure comfort and safety. If you have any health concerns, consult with a qualified yoga instructor or healthcare provider before starting a new practice.

Tai Chi

Tai Chi is a Chinese martial art that emphasizes slow, flowing movements, deep breathing, and mindfulness. Known as "meditation in motion," Tai Chi promotes the smooth flow of Qi and helps balance yin and yang energies. Practicing Tai Chi can improve flexibility, balance, and muscle strength. It also enhances overall well-being and mental clarity, making it beneficial for regulating menstrual cycles and reducing stress.

Here are some Tai Chi movements that can be beneficial for regulating menstrual cycles and promoting reproductive health, along with instructions on how to perform them:

Wave Hands Like Clouds

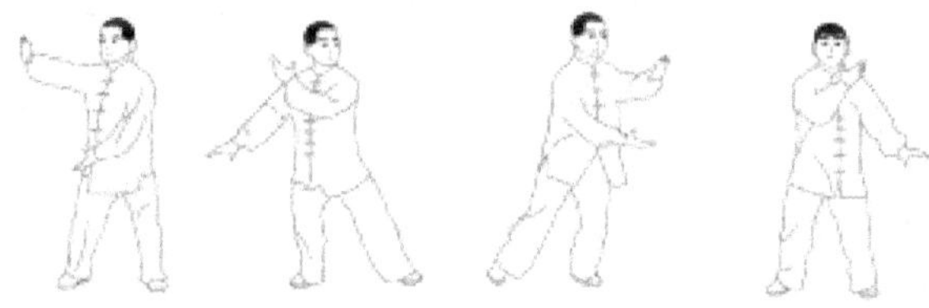

- Stand with your feet shoulder-width apart.
- Begin with your hands in front of your body at chest height.
- Shift your weight to your left foot and turn your upper body slightly to the left.
- Allow your right hand to rise while your left hand lowers, as if you were gently waving your hands in a cloud-like motion.
- Shift your weight to your right foot and turn your upper body to the right, reversing the hand movements.

- Repeat this movement slowly and smoothly for several repetitions.

Grasp Sparrow's Tail

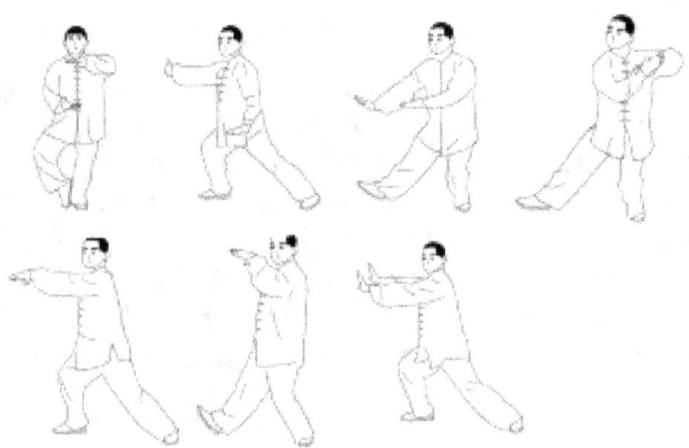

- Start with your feet shoulder-width apart while standing.
- Begin by shifting your weight onto your right foot and stepping back with your left foot.
- Turn your body to the left while extending your left hand forward and pulling your right hand back, as if grasping a sparrow's tail.
- Slowly shift your weight forward and step forward with your left foot.
- Repeat the movement on the other side, shifting your weight onto your left foot and stepping back with your right foot.
- Perform this movement slowly and gracefully for several repetitions.

Parting the Wild Horse's Mane

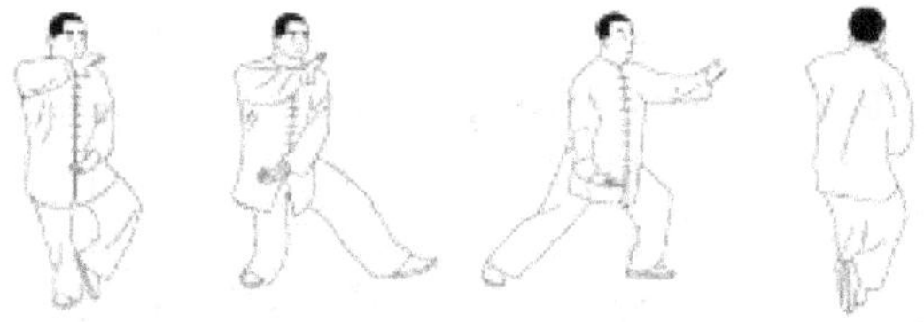

- Stand with your feet shoulder-width apart.
- Shift your weight onto your right foot and step to the left with your left foot.
- As you step, raise your left hand to chest height while your right hand moves down and back.
- Shift your weight onto your left foot and step to the right with your right foot.
- As you step, raise your right hand to chest height while your left hand moves down and back.
- Repeat this movement slowly and smoothly for several repetitions.

These Tai Chi movements can help improve reproductive health by reducing stress, and supporting the flow of Qi throughout the body. Practicing these movements regularly can help regulate menstrual cycles and support overall well-being. If you are new to Tai Chi, consider working with a qualified instructor to ensure you learn the movements correctly and safely.

Qigong

Qigong is another ancient Chinese practice that involves slow, deliberate movements, meditation, and controlled breathing. Qigong aims to cultivate and harmonize Qi within the body, supporting overall health and wellness. For women seeking to regulate their menstrual cycles, Qigong can promote relaxation, improve circulation, and reduce stress levels. Practicing Qigong regularly may also help alleviate PMS and other menstrual-related symptoms.

Governing Vessel Breathing (Ren and Du Channels)

- Stand or sit comfortably with your spine straight.
- Place your hands gently on your lower abdomen.
- Inhale deeply and slowly, directing your breath down into your abdomen.
- Visualize energy flowing up your spine (Du Channel) as you exhale, and then down the front of your body (Ren Channel) as you inhale.
- Repeat this movement for several breaths, focusing on the flow of energy through these channels.

Embracing the Moon

- Stand with your feet shoulder-width apart.
- Begin with your arms extended in front of your body at chest height, palms facing each other.
- Inhale as you slowly open your arms out to the sides, as if you were embracing the moon.
- Exhale as you bring your arms back to the starting position.
- Repeat the movement for several breaths, keeping your movements smooth and gentle.

Gathering Qi from the Heavens

- Stand with your feet shoulder-width apart.
- Begin with your arms at your sides.
- Inhale as you raise your arms slowly above your head, as if gathering Qi from the heavens.
- Exhale as you bring your arms down slowly, guiding the gathered Qi down to your lower abdomen.
- Repeat the movement for several breaths, focusing on the flow of energy.

Circulating Qi in the Lower Abdomen

- Stand with your feet shoulder-width apart.
- Place your hands gently on your lower abdomen.
- Begin by making slow, circular movements with your hands around your lower abdomen.
- Inhale as your hands move upward, and exhale as they move downward.
- Repeat the movement for several breaths, focusing on the flow of energy in your lower abdomen.

Swinging Arm and Breathing

- Stand with your feet shoulder-width apart.
- Allow your arms to hang loosely by your sides.
- Begin swinging your arms gently back and forth while shifting your weight from one foot to the other.
- Breathe naturally and allow the movement to be smooth and rhythmic.
- Continue swinging your arms for several breaths, focusing on relaxation and the flow of energy.

These Qigong movements can help support reproductive health by promoting relaxation, reducing stress, and improving the flow of Qi and blood throughout the body. Practicing Qigong regularly can help regulate menstrual cycles and promote overall well-being. If you are new to Qigong, consider working with a qualified instructor to ensure you learn the movements correctly and safely.

Cultivating Mindfulness for Holistic Wellness

Mindfulness practices play a pivotal role in promoting holistic wellness according to Traditional Chinese Medicine (TCM), offering profound benefits for both physical and mental health. Research has shown that practicing mindfulness can reduce stress, anxiety, and depression, enhance emotional resilience, and improve overall well-being. A study published in the Journal of Alternative and Complementary Medicine (2019) found that mindfulness-based interventions significantly decreased stress levels and improved quality of life in women with menstrual disorders, highlighting the therapeutic potential of mindfulness in women's health.

To cultivate mindfulness and reap its health benefits, consider incorporating the following techniques into your daily routine:

Mindful Breathing

Find a quiet place. Sit or lie down comfortably. Close your eyes and focus on breathing. Notice the sensations of inhalation and exhalation without trying to change them. Allow your breath to flow naturally, focusing on the rise and fall of your abdomen or the sensation of air passing through your nostrils. Gently bring focus back to your breath if your mind wanders. Practice for 5-10 minutes daily.

Body Scan Meditation

Lie down in a comfortable position, close your eyes, and bring your attention to your toes. Slowly scan your body from head to toe, paying attention to any sensations, tension, or discomfort you may encounter. Breathe into each area of your body with awareness, allowing tension to release with each exhale. Spend 5-10 minutes scanning your entire body, observing without judgment.

Mindful Eating

Before eating, take a moment to appreciate the appearance, aroma, and texture of your food. As you eat, chew slowly and mindfully, savoring each bite and paying attention to the flavors and sensations in your mouth. Notice any thoughts or emotions that arise as you eat, and bring your focus back to the present moment if your mind starts to wander. Eating mindfully can enhance digestion, improve satisfaction, and cultivate gratitude for nourishment.

Walking Meditation

Find a quiet outdoor space or walk indoors in a spacious area. Begin walking at a slow, deliberate pace, paying attention to the sensations of each step—the shifting of your weight, the movement of your muscles, and the contact of your feet with the ground. Stay present with each moment of walking, letting go of distractions and thoughts as they arise. Engage your senses fully, noticing the sights, sounds, and smells around you. Walk mindfully for 10-15 minutes, allowing yourself to feel grounded and connected to the present moment

Recommended Ways to Integrate Holistic Wellness into Everyday Living

For women seeking a holistic approach to menstrual health, TCM offers guided routines that combine physical movement, mindfulness practices, and dietary adjustments.

Creating a personalized routine that incorporates TCM principles, exercise, and mindfulness can significantly improve menstrual health. Here are some guided routines for women seeking a holistic approach:

Morning

- Start the day with gentle stretching and deep breathing exercises to wake up the body and mind.
- Practice a few yoga poses such as the cat-cow stretch and the butterfly pose to stimulate the reproductive organs and improve blood flow.

Midday

- Take breaks throughout the day to perform a few minutes of Qi Gong exercises, such as the Eight Brocades, to boost energy and reduce stress.
- Incorporate Tai Chi movements during a lunch break to promote relaxation and mental clarity.

Evening

- Wind down with calming yoga poses like the legs-up-the-wall pose and the supine twist to relax the body and alleviate menstrual discomfort.
- Practice meditation or mindfulness techniques to ease anxiety and improve emotional well-being.

9

Integrating TCM Principles into Modern Living

In today's fast-paced world, integrating Traditional Chinese Medicine (TCM) principles into our daily lives can be a powerful tool for promoting health and well-being amidst the hustle and bustle. While managing hectic schedules and busy routines, it's essential to find practical ways to incorporate TCM practices that support our physical, emotional, and spiritual health. Here are some practical methods for integrating TCM principles into modern living:

Mindful Morning Routine

Starting the day with mindfulness allows you to cultivate awareness of your internal state, connect with the present moment, and set a positive tone for the day ahead. From a TCM perspective, the morning is a time of renewal and regeneration, when the body's Qi (vital energy) is at its peak and primed for nourishment and cultivation.

Engaging in a mindful morning routine can help regulate the flow of Qi and blood, harmonize the organ systems, and promote emotional balance. Begin by practicing gentle stretching or exercises to invigorate the body and cultivate Qi flow. Take a few moments for deep breathing and meditation to calm the mind and center yourself for the day ahead.

TCM-Inspired Nutrition

TCM-inspired nutrition emphasizes the concept of food as medicine, recognizing the profound impact that dietary choices can have on overall health and well-being. Central to TCM dietary principles is the idea of balance and harmony, both within the body and in relation to external factors such as the seasons, climate, and individual constitution. In TCM, each person is believed to have a unique body constitution, influenced by factors such as genetics, lifestyle, and environment. Understanding your constitution is key to making dietary choices that promote health and vitality.

Utilizing the knowledge of TCM, you can tailor your diet to complement their body constitution and address any imbalances or disharmonies within the body. For example, someone with a "Yang" constitution, characterized by warmth, energy, and activity, may benefit from foods that are cooling and nourishing, such as leafy greens, cucumber, and melons, to help balance excess heat and promote a sense of calm and relaxation. Conversely, someone with a "Yin" constitution, characterized by coolness, stillness, and moisture, may benefit from foods that are warming and invigorating, such as ginger, cinnamon, and root vegetables, to help stimulate digestion and circulation.

TCM-inspired nutrition also considers the energetic properties of foods, including their tastes, colors, and textures. According to TCM theory, each taste corresponds to a specific organ system and has unique therapeutic properties. For example, sour foods are believed to tonify the Liver, bitter foods to clear heat and dry dampness, and sweet foods to nourish the Spleen and promote digestion. By incorporating a variety of tastes and textures into the diet, you can support the balance and function of your organ systems and promote overall health and vitality.

Midday Movement Breaks

Midday movement breaks promote the smooth flow of Qi (vital energy) and blood throughout the body, preventing stagnation, and promoting overall health and well-being. Physical movement is essential for maintaining the balance of Yin and Yang energies within the body and harmonizing the organ systems. Midday movement breaks help to invigorate the body's Qi and stimulate circulation, preventing energy blockages and boost vitality.

During midday movement breaks, you can engage in simple exercises and stretches to release tension, improve circulation, and enhance mental clarity. Even in a small space, there are numerous ways to move the body and promote health. Some examples of movement practices suitable for midday breaks include:

Standing or Seated Stretches

Stretching the arms, legs, neck, and spine can help to release tension and improve flexibility. Simple stretches such as reaching overhead, twisting gently from side to side, and folding forward can be performed while standing or sitting in a chair.

Desk Exercises

Simple exercises such as leg lifts, calf raises, and shoulder rolls can be performed discreetly at a desk or workstation. These exercises help to stimulate circulation, prevent stiffness, and improve posture, promoting overall comfort and well-being during the workday.

Mindful Walking

Taking a short walk outdoors or indoors can help to refresh the mind, uplift the spirits, and promote circulation. Mindful walking involves paying attention to each step, feeling the connection with the ground beneath the feet, and appreciating the sights and sounds of the environment.

By incorporating midday movement breaks into your routine, you can support your overall health and well-being, prevent energy stagnation, and enhance productivity and focus throughout the day. These brief moments of movement and mindfulness offer opportunities to recharge the body and mind, fostering balance and harmony in alignment with TCM principles.

Stress Management Strategies

Stress management is particularly important in TCM because it affects the Liver, which is responsible for the smooth flow of Qi and the regulation of emotions. According to TCM principles, emotional stress, frustration, and anger can lead to Liver Qi stagnation, resulting in symptoms such as irritability, mood swings, and tension in the body. Over time, unresolved stress can also impact other organ systems, leading to a cascade of imbalances and health issues.

In addition to its effects on the Liver, stress can also weaken the Spleen, which governs digestion and the transformation of food into Qi and blood. Chronic stress can impair spleen function, leading to symptoms such as poor appetite, fatigue, and digestive disturbances. By managing stress effectively, you can support the balance and function of the Liver and Spleen, promote the smooth flow of Qi and blood, and enhance overall health and well-being.

Incorporating short mindfulness practices, such as deep breathing exercises or mindful walking breaks, can help to calm the mind, reduce tension, and promote mental clarity. Taking regular breaks to stretch or engage in gentle movement can alleviate physical tension and improve circulation, while practicing gratitude or visualization techniques can shift focus away from stressors and foster a positive mindset. Setting boundaries, prioritizing tasks, and practicing time management techniques can also help to reduce overwhelm and create a sense of control amidst a busy schedule. Finally, connecting with supportive friends or loved ones, seeking professional support when needed, and fostering self-compassion and acceptance are valuable strategies for navigating stress in modern life.

Evening Rituals for Relaxation

Create evening rituals that promote relaxation and restful sleep. Wind down with a warm bath infused with aromatic herbs or essential oils to soothe tired muscles and calm the mind. Enjoy a cup of chamomile or lavender tea to promote relaxation and prepare the body for restorative sleep. Limit screen time before bed and engage in calming activities such as reading or gentle stretching to signal to the body that it's time to unwind.

Integrating TCM Modalities

Explore integrative approaches to health and well-being by incorporating TCM modalities such as acupuncture, herbal medicine, or energy healing into your wellness routine. Schedule regular appointments with qualified practitioners to address specific health concerns and maintain balance within the body. Be proactive in seeking support and guidance from healthcare professionals who align with your holistic health goals.

Cultivating Connection to Nature

Connect with the natural world to replenish your Qi and nourish your spirit. Spend time outdoors in green spaces, parks, or natural environments to ground yourself and absorb the healing energies of nature. Practice earthing techniques such as walking barefoot or gardening to harmonize with the Earth's energy and promote overall well-being.

By integrating these practical methods into your day-to-day life, you can harness the wisdom of TCM to navigate modern living with greater ease, resilience, and vitality. By prioritizing self-care, mindfulness, and balance, you can cultivate a holistic approach to health that supports your well-being on all levels. Remember that small, consistent changes can lead to significant transformations over time, and finding harmony amidst the busyness of life is both achievable and empowering.

10

Finding Your Flow: Supporting Menstrual Harmony Through Balance

In the final chapter of "From Qi to Flow: Adapting Wisdom of Traditional Chinese Medicine to Regulate Menstrual Cycle," we delve into essential practices for nurturing balance and promoting menstrual wellness. Drawing on the principles of Traditional Chinese Medicine (TCM), we explore how prioritizing rest and sleep, tracking your cycle, maintaining a healthy weight, and seeking support and guidance can play crucial roles in restoring harmony to the body and mind. By integrating these holistic practices into your daily routine, you can cultivate a deeper understanding of your body's rhythms and empower yourself to achieve optimal menstrual health.

In the following sections, we will delve into each of these practices through the lens of TCM, examining why they are important for supporting the body's natural healing processes and promoting overall well-being. From the restorative power of sleep to the insights gained from cycle tracking, each practice offers valuable opportunities for self-care and self-discovery. Let us embark on this journey together, as we uncover the transformative potential of nurturing balance in our lives and embracing the wisdom of TCM for menstrual wellness.

Prioritize Rest and Sleep

Sleep is considered a crucial time for the body to replenish Yin essence and nourish the blood, both of which are essential for a healthy menstrual cycle. During sleep, the body enters a state of deep rest and restoration, allowing Qi to flow smoothly and harmoniously throughout the meridians. When we prioritize adequate rest and sleep, we support the body's ability to maintain balance and harmony, which in turn promotes regularity and ease in the menstrual cycle.

Insufficient rest and sleep can lead to imbalances in the body's energy systems, particularly affecting the Liver and Spleen meridians, which are closely involved in menstrual health. According to TCM principles, Liver Qi stagnation and Spleen deficiency are common patterns associated with irregular menstruation, menstrual pain, and other menstrual disorders. By ensuring adequate rest and sleep, we help to regulate the flow of Qi and prevent stagnation, while also supporting the Spleen's ability to transform and transport nutrients and fluids throughout the body. In this way, prioritizing rest and sleep plays a crucial role in maintaining overall balance and vitality, thereby preventing pain and illnesses associated with menstrual irregularities.

Track Your Cycle

Tracking one's menstrual cycle is important for several reasons. Firstly, it provides valuable insight into the body's natural rhythms and patterns, allowing you to identify any deviations or irregularities that may indicate underlying imbalances. By tracking the length of the menstrual cycle, the duration of menstruation, and the quality of menstrual blood, you can gain a deeper understanding of your overall reproductive health and vitality.

Secondly, the menstrual cycle is closely linked to the flow of Qi and Blood within the body, as well as the balance of Yin and Yang energies. By observing changes in menstrual symptoms and sensations throughout the cycle, you can discern patterns of disharmony or stagnation that may be affecting your health. For example, irregular periods, menstrual pain, or changes in the color or consistency of menstrual blood can indicate imbalances in specific organ systems, such as the Liver, Spleen, or Kidneys.

It also enables you to work proactively with TCM practitioners to address any imbalances and restore harmony to the body. By providing detailed information about menstrual symptoms, cycle length, and overall health status, you can receive personalized recommendations for herbal remedies, dietary adjustments, and acupuncture treatments, as well as lifestyle modifications tailored to your specific needs. This way, tracking the menstrual cycle empowers you to take an active role in your health and well-being, facilitating early intervention and prevention of menstrual disorders and promoting optimal reproductive health from a TCM perspective.

Maintain a Healthy Weight

Maintaining a healthy weight is very important for regulating the menstrual cycle and preventing menstruation-related disorders. According to TCM principles, excess weight can lead to the accumulation of Dampness and Phlegm in the body, which can obstruct the flow of Qi and blood, particularly in the lower abdomen and pelvic region. This obstruction can manifest as irregular menstruation, heavy periods, or menstrual pain due to stagnation and blockages within the channels and meridians.

TCM views the Spleen and Kidneys as key organs responsible for the transformation and transportation of nutrients and fluids throughout the body. Excess weight can place strain on these organs, leading to Spleen deficiency and Kidney Yang deficiency, which are common patterns associated with menstrual irregularities. Spleen deficiency can impair the

Spleen's ability to regulate the menstrual cycle, while Kidney Yang deficiency can weaken the Kidneys' capacity to support reproductive function and hormonal balance.

By maintaining a healthy weight, you can support the smooth flow of Qi and blood, optimize the function of the spleen and Kidneys, and promote overall balance and harmony within the body. This, in turn, helps to regulate the menstrual cycle, alleviate menstrual disorders, and prevent the accumulation of Dampness and Phlegm that can contribute to menstrual pain and discomfort. Through a combination of dietary modifications, regular exercise, and lifestyle adjustments, you can work towards achieving a healthy weight and supporting optimal reproductive health.

Seek Support and Guidance

Navigating your menstrual wellness journey can be challenging, but you don't have to do it alone. Seek support from a qualified TCM practitioner, healthcare provider, or support group to help you along the way. They can offer personalized advice and guidance tailored to your unique needs.

By following these practical tips and incorporating TCM principles into your lifestyle, you can create a personalized plan for maintaining menstrual wellness. Remember, each journey is unique, so be patient and persistent as you work towards achieving optimal health and balance.

Case Studies

Jane's Journey with Endometriosis and Traditional Chinese Medicine

Background

Jane, a 32-year-old professional living in a busy urban environment, was diagnosed with endometriosis in her late twenties after experiencing intense menstrual cramps and heavy bleeding. Her body constitution was described as being prone to cold and dampness, and she often felt fatigued and bloated. Prior to learning about Traditional Chinese Medicine (TCM), Jane's dietary habits included consuming a lot of cold and raw foods, such as salads and smoothies, which exacerbated her internal coldness. She also had a high intake of processed foods and caffeine.

Introduction to TCM

Frustrated with the side effects and limited relief from conventional treatments, Jane sought out alternative options. She learned about TCM from a friend who had benefited from acupuncture for a different health issue. Intrigued, Jane decided to visit a TCM practitioner specializing in women's health.

TCM Treatment Approach

The TCM practitioner assessed Jane's overall health and identified an imbalance in her body related to cold, dampness, and Qi stagnation. The practitioner proposed a holistic treatment plan that included dietary modifications, herbal medicine, acupuncture, and acupressure.

1. **Dietary Modifications:**
- Jane was advised to reduce her intake of cold and raw foods, focusing instead on warming and cooked meals.

- She incorporated more warming spices like ginger and cinnamon into her diet and avoided cold drinks and excess caffeine.

- Jane also increased her consumption of nourishing soups and broths.

2. **Herbal Medicine:**
- The practitioner prescribed Jane an herbal formula, "Si Wu Tang" (Four-Substance Decoction), known to nourish blood and improve circulation.

3. **Acupuncture and Acupressure:**
- Jane underwent regular acupuncture sessions targeting specific meridian points associated with reproductive health.

- The practitioner taught Jane acupressure techniques to use at home to manage pain and promote circulation.

4. **Lifestyle Adjustments:**
- Jane's practitioner recommended her to incorporate stress-reducing activities such as meditation in addition to 20 minutes of gentle exercise (such as yoga or qigong).

- Prioritizing adequate sleep and establishing a regular sleep schedule was emphasized to support hormonal balance and overall well-being.

- To counterbalance her cold constitution, Jane was advised to take 15 minutes of warm bath daily. It was suggested that she put a tablespoon of Epsom salt into the bathwater to keep the water warmer for longer.

Outcome and Recovery

Jane followed the TCM treatment plan diligently, making significant changes to her diet and lifestyle. After a few months, she noticed a reduction in the severity of her menstrual cramps and overall discomfort. Over the next year, her symptoms continued to improve, and her menstrual cycle became more regular.

By the end of the year, Jane's endometriosis had significantly improved, and her quality of life had dramatically increased. She no longer experienced the intense pain and heavy bleeding she once endured, and she felt more energized and balanced.

Jane's journey with TCM highlights the potential benefits of adopting a holistic approach to treating endometriosis. By addressing her body constitution, making dietary changes, and following a tailored TCM treatment plan, Jane was able to successfully manage and improve her condition. Her experience underscores the value of exploring alternative approaches to women's health issues, particularly for those seeking relief from chronic conditions.

Sarah's Journey with PCOS and Traditional Chinese Medicine

Background

Sarah, a 28-year-old marketing professional, was diagnosed with polycystic ovary syndrome (PCOS) in her early twenties. She experienced irregular menstrual cycles, weight gain, and acne. Her body constitution was described as being prone to dampness and phlegm, which affected her metabolism and hormonal balance. Sarah's dietary habits prior to learning about Traditional Chinese Medicine (TCM) included a high intake of processed foods and refined sugars. She often skipped meals due to her busy schedule and relied on coffee and energy drinks to stay awake.

Introduction to TCM

After struggling with her PCOS symptoms for years and experiencing limited success with conventional treatments, Sarah sought alternative options. She learned about TCM through online research and testimonials from women who had benefited from it for various health issues. Intrigued, Sarah decided to visit a TCM practitioner who specialized in women's health and hormonal imbalances.

TCM Treatment Approach

The TCM practitioner assessed Sarah's overall health and identified an imbalance in her body related to dampness and phlegm stagnation, as well as liver Qi stagnation. The practitioner proposed a holistic treatment plan that included dietary modifications, herbal medicine, acupuncture, and acupressure.

1. Dietary Modifications

- Sarah was advised to avoid processed foods and refined sugars, focusing instead on whole, unprocessed foods.

- She incorporated more warming foods like ginger, cinnamon, and cooked vegetables into her diet.

- Sarah was also encouraged to eat regular meals and include protein-rich foods to stabilize her blood sugar levels.

2. Herbal Medicine

- The practitioner prescribed an herbal formula, "Gui Zhi Fu Ling Wan" (Cinnamon and Poria Pill), known for promoting blood circulation and removing dampness and phlegm

3. Acupuncture and Acupressure

- Sarah underwent regular acupuncture sessions targeting specific meridian points associated with PCOS symptoms and hormonal balance.

- The practitioner taught Sarah acupressure techniques she could use at home to manage symptoms and improve energy flow.

4. Acupuncture and Acupressure

- Sarah underwent regular acupuncture sessions targeting specific meridian points associated with PCOS symptoms and hormonal balance.

- The practitioner taught Sarah acupressure techniques she could use at home to manage symptoms and improve energy flow.

5. Lifestyle Adjustments

- Sarah was advised to incorporate stress reducing activities such as short sessions of deep breathing, and meditation into her daily routine to reduce the impact of stress on her hormonal balance.

- Daily physical activity, such as walking, tai chi and yoga, was recommended to improve insulin sensitivity, promote weight management and support overall health.

- Prioritizing adequate sleep and establishing a regular sleep schedule was emphasized to support hormonal balance and overall well-being.

Outcome and Recovery

Sarah followed the TCM treatment plan consistently and made significant changes to her diet and lifestyle. After a few months, she noticed improvements in her menstrual cycle regularity and a reduction in acne and weight gain. Her energy levels also improved, and she felt more balanced overall.

Over the course of a year, Sarah's PCOS symptoms continued to improve, and she achieved more consistent menstrual cycles without any hormonal medications. Her overall quality of life improved significantly, and she felt more in control of her health.

Sarah's journey with TCM showcases the potential benefits of a
holistic approach to treating PCOS. By addressing her body
constitution, making dietary changes, and following a tailored
TCM treatment plan, Sarah was able to successfully manage and
improve her condition. Her experience highlights the value of
exploring alternative approaches for women's health issues,
particularly for those seeking relief from chronic conditions like
PCOS.

Emily's Journey to Conception with Traditional Chinese Medicine

Background

Emily, a 34-year-old teacher, had experienced recurrent
miscarriages, which left her feeling devastated and unsure of
what steps to take next. After her third miscarriage, she sought
medical advice and was told there was no clear explanation for
the losses. Emily's body constitution was described as having a
deficiency in Kidney essence and spleen Qi, which affected her
fertility and ability to sustain a pregnancy. Prior to learning
about Traditional Chinese Medicine (TCM), Emily's dietary
habits included a preference for cold foods and raw salads,
which contributed to internal coldness.

Introduction to TCM

In her quest for answers and potential solutions, Emily began
researching alternative approaches and discovered TCM. She
found several success stories of women who had faced similar
challenges and overcame them with the help of TCM. Intrigued,
Emily decided to visit a TCM practitioner who specialized in
fertility and women's health.

TCM Treatment Approach

The TCM practitioner conducted a thorough assessment of
Emily's overall health and identified imbalances in her Kidney
essence and spleen Qi. The practitioner proposed a holistic

treatment plan that included dietary modifications, herbal medicine, and acupuncture to strengthen her reproductive system and address her deficiencies.

1. Dietary Modifications
- Emily was advised to avoid cold and raw foods, focusing instead on warm and cooked meals to nurture her body.

- She was encouraged to eat nutrient-dense foods such as soups, stews, and warming herbs like ginger and cinnamon.

- Emily also increased her intake of foods that support Kidney health, such as black beans and walnuts.

2. Herbal Medicine
- The practitioner prescribed an herbal formula, "Si Wu Tang" (Four-Substance Decoction), known for nourishing the blood and improving circulation.

3. Acupuncture
- Emily underwent regular acupuncture sessions targeting meridian points associated with fertility and reproductive health.

- The practitioner focused on improving circulation and supporting the Kidney and Spleen functions.

4. Lifestyle Adjustments
- Emily was recommended to incorporate stress-reducing activities such as mindfulness meditation and deep breathing exercises into her daily routine.
- Engaging in regular physical activity, such as walking, and yoga for at least 20 minutes a day was advised to improve blood circulation and reduce stress.

Outcome and Recovery

Emily diligently followed the TCM treatment plan, making significant changes to her diet and lifestyle. After six months of treatment, Emily's overall health improved, and she noticed a more regular menstrual cycle and fewer symptoms of fatigue.

After about a year of consistent treatment and care, Emily became pregnant again. This time, she experienced a smooth pregnancy and delivered a healthy baby nine months later. Emily attributes her successful pregnancy to the holistic approach of TCM, which strengthened her reproductive system and supported her journey to motherhood.

Emily's journey with TCM demonstrates the potential benefits of a holistic approach to fertility issues, particularly for women experiencing recurrent miscarriages. By addressing her body constitution, making dietary changes, and following a tailored TCM treatment plan, Emily was able to successfully conceive and carry a healthy pregnancy to term. Her experience underscores the value of exploring alternative approaches to women's health challenges and the importance of personalized care.

Conclusion

In concluding this book, it is essential to acknowledge the profound wisdom of Traditional Chinese Medicine (TCM) in guiding us towards optimal menstrual health and well-being. Throughout these pages, we have explored the intricate connections between the body, mind, and spirit, recognizing that our menstrual cycles are not separate from but deeply intertwined with our overall health and vitality. TCM teaches us to view menstruation not as a burden to endure but as a natural process to embrace, offering us insights and tools to navigate our menstrual wellness with grace and empowerment.

At the heart of TCM philosophy lies the belief in the body's innate ability to heal itself from within. By harmonizing the flow of Qi, balancing the forces of Yin and Yang, and nourishing the Blood and Essence, TCM facilitates the body's natural healing processes, enabling us to overcome imbalances and restore equilibrium to our menstrual cycles. While TCM offers valuable guidance and support, it is ultimately the body's wisdom and resilience that drive the journey towards healing and wellness.

As we bid farewell to these pages, it is my sincerest wish that the knowledge and practices shared in this book serve as a beacon of light and hope for all readers. May you find solace in knowing that you are not alone in your journey towards menstrual wellness, and that there are gentle yet powerful tools at your disposal to alleviate discomfort, pain, and imbalances that may arise during menstruation. May you embrace your menstrual cycle as a sacred and natural aspect of your being, honoring its rhythms and messages with compassion and understanding.

May this book empower you to listen to your body's whispers, to nourish yourself with kindness and self-care, and to cultivate a deep sense of connection and harmony within. May you find joy and vitality in every phase of your menstrual cycle, celebrating its cyclical nature as a reflection of the ebb and flow of life itself. And may you carry forth the wisdom of TCM with you, sharing it with others and spreading the seeds of healing and transformation far and wide.

As we embark on the journey ahead, let us remember that true wellness is not merely the absence of illness, but a state of vibrant health, balance, and wholeness in body, mind, and spirit. May you embody this vision of wellness in all aspects of your life, and may your menstrual cycles be a source of strength, vitality, and empowerment for years to come.

Appendix A

Resources Used for Reference

Books and Authors

1. Williams, Tom. *Chinese Medicine: A Comprehensive System for Health and Fitness.* Weatherhill, 1995.
2. Beinfield, Harriet, and Efrem Korngold. *Between Heaven and Earth: A Guide to Chinese Medicine.* Ballantine Books, 1992.
3. Deadman, Peter, Mazin Al-Khafaji, and Kevin Baker. *A Manual of Acupuncture.* Journal of Chinese Medicine Publications, 2007.
4. Harriet, H. and Korngold, E. *Between Heaven and Earth: A Guide to Chinese Medicine.* Ballantine Books, 1992.
5. Kaptchuk, Ted J. *The Web That Has No Weaver: Understanding Chinese Medicine.* Contemporary Books, 2000.
6. Elias, J and Ketcham, K. *Chinese Medicine for Maximum Immunity: Understanding the Five Elemental Types for Health and Well-Being.* Healing Arts Press, 1998.
7. Lyttleton, Jane. *Treating Infertility with Traditional Chinese Medicine.* Churchill Livingston, Inc., 2013.
8. Lo, Chi Chiu, and Ganglin Yin. *Acupuncture and Chinese Herbal Medicine for Women's Health: Bridging the Gap Between Western and Eastern Medicine.* Singing Dragon, 2016.
9. Maciocia, G. *Obstetrics and Gynecology in Chinese Medicine.* Churchill Livingstone, 2011.
10. Randall, V. and Gu, S. *Traditional Chinese Medicine: Scientific Basis for Its Use.* Royal Society of Chemistry, 2013.
11. Reid, Daniel P. *The Complete Book of Chinese Health & Healing: Guarding the Three Treasures.* Shambhala, 1995.
12. Ross, Jeremy. *The Fertile Soul: Ten Ancient Chinese Secrets to Tap into a Woman's Creative Potential.* Harper Collins, 2007.

13. Liu, Liang and Liu, Zhanwen. *Essentials of Chinese Medicine: Volume 1*. Springer Science & Business Media, 2010.
14. Valaskova, K. *The Secrets of Chinese Medicine: A Complete Guide to the Principles and Practices of Traditional Chinese Medicine*. Independently Published, 2019.
15. Wiseman, Nigel, and Andy Ellis. *Fundamentals of Chinese Medicine*. Paradigm Publications, 1995.
16. Xuemin, Shi, and Zhao Zhang. *An Illustrated Handbook of Chinese Medicine*. Foreign Languages Press, 1993.
17. Yang, Shou-Zhong. *The Divine Farmer's Materia Medica: A Translation of the Shen Nong Ben Cao*. Blue Poppy Enterprises, Inc., 1998.
18. Yeung, Him-Che. *Handbook of Chinese Herbs and Formulas*. Institute of Chinese Medicine, 1985.
19. Zhang, Enqin. *A Practical English-Chinese Library of Traditional Chinese Medicine (Volume 1: Basic Theory)*. Shanghai Scientific & Technical Publishers, 1995.
20. Dan, Bensky. *Chinese Herbal Medicine: Materia Medica*. Eastland Press, 2015.

Studies

1. Chen, L., & Chen, W. (2017). Effects of acupuncture and moxibustion in patients with polycystic ovary syndrome: A systematic review and meta-analysis. *Journal of Traditional Chinese Medicine,* 37(5), 646-653.
2. Li, X., & Liu, H. (2018). A systematic review and meta-analysis of Chinese herbal medicine in the treatment of primary dysmenorrhea. *Evidence-Based Complementary and Alternative Medicine,* 2018, 1-15.
3. Liu, Y., Ma, H., & Wang, L. (2019). Chinese herbal medicine for premenstrual syndrome: A systematic review and meta-analysis of randomized controlled trials. *Complementary Therapies in Medicine,* 44, 181-188.
4. Park, J., & Kim, D. (2016). Efficacy and safety of traditional herbal medicine for the treatment of primary dysmenorrhea: A

systematic review and meta-analysis. *Evidence-Based Complementary and Alternative Medicine, 2016, 1-10.*

5. Song, H., & Xue, Q. (2018). Effects of traditional Chinese medicine on menstrual irregularities: A meta-analysis of randomized controlled trials. *Journal of Integrative Medicine, 16(3),* 147-154.

6. Wang, S., & Li, D. (2017). Acupuncture for menstrual pain: A systematic review and meta-analysis of randomized controlled trials. *Journal of Alternative and Complementary Medicine, 23(5),* 336-345.

7. Xu, Q., & Jiang, Y. (2019). The efficacy and safety of Chinese herbal medicine for the treatment of primary dysmenorrhea: A systematic review and meta-analysis. *Evidence-Based Complementary and Alternative Medicine, 2019,* 1-15.

8. Yang, J., & Wu, C. (2018). A systematic review and meta-analysis of the efficacy of acupuncture in the treatment of primary dysmenorrhea. *Journal of Alternative and Complementary Medicine, 24(3),* 206-217.

9. Zhang, Y., & Li, H. (2016). Chinese herbal medicine for primary dysmenorrhea: A systematic review and meta-analysis of randomized controlled trials. *Journal of Ethnopharmacology,* 183, 159-167.

10. Chen, X., & Wang, Y. (2017). Efficacy and safety of Kampo medicine for the treatment of menstrual irregularities: A systematic review and meta-analysis. *Phytotherapy Research,* 31(9), 1317-1326.

11. Dong, J., & Wang, W. (2018). Effects of Kampo medicine on menstrual pain: A meta-analysis of randomized controlled trials. *Evidence-Based Complementary and Alternative Medicine,* 2018, 1-10.

12. Han, L., & Liu, S. (2019). The efficacy of Kampo medicine for the treatment of primary dysmenorrhea: A systematic review and meta-analysis of randomized controlled trials. *Journal of Integrative Medicine,* 17(4), 251-259.

13. Hirata, K., & Ishikawa, S. (2017). A systematic review and meta-analysis of Kampo medicine for menstrual irregularities: The evidence from randomized controlled trials. *Complementary Therapies in Medicine,* 33, 82-89.

14. Hu, J., & Chen, Y. (2018). Efficacy and safety of Kampo medicine for primary dysmenorrhea: A systematic review and

meta-analysis of randomized controlled trials. *Journal of Ethnopharmacology,* 227, 164-175.

15. Itoh, T., & Sato, Y. (2016). The effectiveness of Kampo medicine for menstrual pain: A meta-analysis of randomized controlled trials. *Evidence-Based Complementary and Alternative Medicine,* 2016, 1-11.

16. Kim, S., & Park, S. (2018). A systematic review and meta-analysis of Kampo medicine for primary dysmenorrhea: The evidence from randomized controlled trials. *Journal of Alternative and Complementary Medicine,* 24(7), 622-632.

17. Lee, J., & Lee, S. (2017). Effects of Kampo medicine on menstrual irregularities: A meta-analysis of randomized controlled trials. *Journal of Ethnopharmacology,* 195, 207-214.

18. Miyakawa, Y., & Yamada, T. (2019). The efficacy and safety of Kampo medicine for the treatment of primary dysmenorrhea: A systematic review and meta-analysis of randomized controlled trials. *Complementary Therapies in Medicine,* 43, 103-111.

19. Nakamura, T., & Hoshino, T. (2018). A systematic review and meta-analysis of Kampo medicine for menstrual pain: The evidence from randomized controlled trials. *Journal of Integrative Medicine,* 16(5), 322-331.

20. Ogura-Tsujita, Y., & Yamaguchi, R. (2017). The effectiveness of Kampo medicine for menstrual irregularities: A meta-analysis of randomized controlled trials. *Complementary Therapies in Medicine,* 32, 40-45.

21. Tanaka, M., & Kobayashi, N. (2018). Effects of Kampo medicine on menstrual pain: A systematic review and meta-analysis of randomized controlled trials. *Journal of Alternative and Complementary Medicine,* 24(10), 965-974.

22. Zhang, Y., & Liu, J. (2019). A systematic review and meta-analysis of Kampo medicine for primary dysmenorrhea: The evidence from randomized controlled trials. *Evidence-Based Complementary and Alternative Medicine,* 2019, 1-14.

Websites

1. **Acupuncture.com**

   acupuncture.com

   Acupuncture.com offers a comprehensive resource on acupuncture, Chinese medicine, and related modalities. It features articles, forums, and educational materials for practitioners and patients alike.

2. **American Herbalists Guild (AHG)**

   americanherbalistsguild.com

   The AHG is a professional organization dedicated to promoting the practice of herbal medicine in the United States. Its website provides educational resources, practitioner directories, and information on herbalism and botanical medicine.

3. **Blue Poppy Enterprises, Inc.**

   bluepoppy.com

   Blue Poppy Enterprises is a leading publisher of books, educational materials, and herbal products in the field of Traditional Chinese Medicine. Its website offers a wide range of resources for students, practitioners, and enthusiasts of TCM.

4. **Chinese Medicine Living**

   chinesemedicineliving.com

   Chinese Medicine Living is an online platform dedicated to exploring the principles and practices of Traditional Chinese Medicine. It features articles, recipes, and resources for promoting health and wellness through TCM.

5. **National Certification Commission for Acupuncture and Oriental Medicine (NCCAOM)**

nccaom.org

Description: The NCCAOM is a nonprofit organization that certifies acupuncturists and Oriental medicine practitioners in the United States. Its website offers information on certification requirements, continuing education, and professional standards in the field of acupuncture and Oriental medicine.

6. **National Institutes of Health (NIH) - Office of Dietary Supplements (ODS)**

ods.od.nih.gov

The ODS provides evidence-based information on dietary supplements, vitamins, and minerals. Its website offers fact sheets, research summaries, and consumer guides to promote informed decision-making about dietary supplement use.

7. **Qi Journal**

qi-journal.com

Description: Qi Journal is an online publication dedicated to exploring the principles and practices of Qigong, Tai Chi, acupuncture, and Chinese medicine. It features articles, interviews, and resources for enthusiasts of Chinese martial arts and holistic health.

8. **Shen-Nong Limited**

shen-nong.com

Description: Shen-Nong Limited is a leading provider of information on Chinese herbs and traditional medicine. Its website offers a comprehensive database of Chinese herbs, formulas, and therapeutic applications.

Appendix B Glossary

Acupuncture: A traditional Chinese medical practice involving the insertion of thin needles into specific points on the body to stimulate energy flow and promote healing.

Ba Zhen Tang: See *Eight Treasures Decoction*

Bai Shao (*Paeonia lactiflora*)**:** A medicinal herb used in Traditional Chinese Medicine to nourish blood, alleviate pain, and promote relaxation.

Bladder: One of the five organs in Traditional Chinese Medicine, responsible for storing and excreting urine and regulating water metabolism.

Blood: A vital substance in the body according to Traditional Chinese Medicine, responsible for nourishing organs, tissues, and cells.

Bupleurum: A medicinal herb used in Traditional Chinese Medicine to relieve liver stagnation, reduce inflammation, and support liver function.

Buplerum and Peony Combination: A traditional Chinese herbal formula consisting of Bupleurum (Chai Hu), Peony (Bai Shao), Dong Quai (Dang Gui), Cinnamon Twig (Gui Zhi), Ginger (Sheng Jiang), and Licorice (Gan Cao). It is commonly used to soothe Liver Qi stagnation, regulate menstruation, and alleviate symptoms such as irregular periods, abdominal pain, and emotional fluctuations.

Cinnamon Twig and Poria Decoction: A decoction made with Cinnamon Twig (Gui Zhi) and Poria (Fu Ling) as its main ingredients, along with other herbs such as Peony Root (Bai

Shao) and Ginger (Sheng Jiang). Used for regulating menstruation and relieving menstrual pain.

Cooling: the ability of certain herbs, foods, and practices to reduce internal heat, clear excess fire, and promote balance and harmony within the body.

Dang Gui (*Angelica sinensis*): Also known as Dong Quai, a popular medicinal herb in Traditional Chinese Medicine used to regulate menstrual cycles, tonify blood, and promote overall vitality.

Dang Gui and Peony Powder: A traditional Chinese herbal formula consisting of Angelica sinensis (Dang Gui) and White Peony Root (Bai Shao). It is commonly used to nourish Blood, regulate menstruation, alleviate menstrual pain, and tonify the Liver and Kidneys in women's health, while also addressing symptoms such as irregular periods, abdominal cramps, and fatigue.

Dang Gui Shao Yao San: See *Dang Gui and Peony Powder*

Decoction: A method of preparing herbal medicine by boiling a combination of herbs in water to extract their active ingredients.

Edema: A condition characterized by the accumulation of excess fluid in the tissues due to weakened Spleen Qi, Kidney Yang deficiency, or obstruction of the channels, often manifesting as swelling, heaviness, and puffiness.

Eight Treasures Decoction: A traditional Chinese herbal formula consisting of Rehmannia (Shu Di Huang), Dioscorea (Shan Yao), Cornus (Shan Zhu Yu), Moutan (Mu Dan Pi), Poria (Fu Ling), Cinnamon Twig (Gui Zhi), Alisma (Ze Xie), and Hoelen (Fu Ling). It is commonly used to nourish the Yin, tonify the Kidneys, and regulate menstruation and hormonal balance in women's health.

Energy: The vital force or life energy that flows through the body according to Traditional Chinese Medicine, influencing health and well-being.

Essence: A fundamental substance in the body according to Traditional Chinese Medicine, encompassing Jing, Qi, and Shen, and representing the foundation of life.

Five Elements: The five elemental energies—Wood, Fire, Earth, Metal, and Water—used in Traditional Chinese Medicine to describe the relationships between various aspects of nature and the human body.

Four Substance Decoction: A traditional Chinese herbal formula consisting of four herbs: Dang Gui (Angelica sinensis), Shu Di Huang (Rehmannia glutinosa), Bai Shao (Paeonia lactiflora), and Chuan Xiong (Ligusticum chuanxiong). Commonly used in Traditional Chinese Medicine to nourish the blood, regulate menstruation, and treat gynecological disorders.

Four Substance Decoction with Peach Pit: A traditional Chinese herbal formula consisting of Persica (Tao Ren), Angelica Sinensis (Dang Gui), Paeonia Lactiflora (Bai Shao), and Atractylodes (Bai Zhu). It is commonly used to invigorate blood circulation, regulate menstruation, and alleviate symptoms such as menstrual pain, irregular periods, and uterine fibroids in women's health.

Fu: The Yang organs, which include the Gallbladder, Stomach, Small Intestine, Large Intestine, Urinary Bladder, and San Jiao (Triple Burner). These organs are responsible for transforming and transporting substances throughout the body, as well as storing waste products before elimination.

Ginger (*Zingiber Officinate*): A medicinal herb used in both Traditional Chinese Medicine and Western herbalism to promote digestion, reduce inflammation, and alleviate nausea.

Gui Zhi Fu Ling Tang: *See Cinnamon Twig and Poria Decoction*

Herbal Medicine: The use of medicinal plants and herbs to prevent and treat various health conditions, practiced in both Traditional Chinese Medicine and other healing systems.

Hormones: Chemical messengers produced by the endocrine system that regulate various bodily functions, including growth, metabolism, and reproduction.

Jia Wei Xiao Yao San: *See Buplerum Peony Combination*

Jing: Also known as Essence, a fundamental substance in Traditional Chinese Medicine representing the body's vitality, essence, and reproductive potential.

Kidney: One of the five organs in Traditional Chinese Medicine, responsible for storing Jing, regulating water metabolism, and supporting reproductive health.

Liu Wei Di Huang Tang: *See Six Flavor Rehmannia Decoction*

Liver: One of the five organs in Traditional Chinese Medicine, responsible for storing blood, regulating Qi flow, and detoxifying the body.

Luteal Phase: The second half of the menstrual cycle, characterized by the release of progesterone and the preparation of the uterine lining for potential implantation.

Menstruation: The monthly shedding of the uterine lining, accompanied by bleeding, signaling the end of the menstrual cycle.

Meridians: Pathways in the body through which Qi (vital energy) flows according to Traditional Chinese Medicine theory. These channels connect various organs, tissues, and functions, influencing health and well-being.

Moxibustion: A Traditional Chinese Medicine therapy involving the burning of mugwort herb to stimulate acupuncture points and promote healing.

Ovulation: The release of a mature egg from the ovary, typically occurring midway through the menstrual cycle.

Peony: A medicinal herb used in Traditional Chinese Medicine to nourish blood, alleviate pain, and promote relaxation.

Qi: Also spelled as Chi, the vital energy or life force that flows through the body according to Traditional Chinese Medicine, influencing health, vitality, and well-being.

Qigong: A mind-body practice involving coordinated movements, breathing exercises, and meditation to cultivate Qi flow, promote health, and harmonize the body and mind.

Rehmannia and Multi Seeds Decoction: A traditional Chinese herbal formula consisting of Rehmannia (Shu Di Huang), Dodder Seed (Tu Si Zi), Plantain Seed (Che Qian Zi), Lycium Fruit (Gou Qi Zi), and Yam Rhizome (Shan Yao). It is commonly used to nourish Yin, tonify the Kidneys, and regulate menstruation and hormonal balance in women's health, while also supporting kidney function, enhancing vision, and promoting overall vitality.

Shen: The spirit or consciousness according to Traditional Chinese Medicine, encompassing mental, emotional, and spiritual aspects of health.

Si Wu Tang: See *Four Substance Decoction*

Six Flavor Rehmannia Decoction: A traditional Chinese herbal formula consisting of Rehmannia (Shu Di Huang), Cornus (Shan Zhu Yu), Dioscorea (Shan Yao), Moutan (Mu Dan Pi), Poria (Fu Ling), and Alisma (Ze Xie). It is commonly used to nourish Yin, tonify the Kidneys, and regulate menstruation and hormonal balance, while also addressing symptoms such as fatigue, dizziness, and lower back pain.

Sheng Di Huang: (*Rehmannia glutinosa):* A medicinal herb used in Traditional Chinese Medicine to tonify Yin, nourish blood, and support Kidney function.

Shu Di Huang: (*Rehmannia glutinosa*, Prepared Rehmannia Root): A commonly used herb in traditional Chinese medicine known for its ability to nourish Yin, tonify the Kidneys, and replenish blood. Unlike Sheng Di Huang, which is the raw form of Rehmannia Root, Shu Di Huang undergoes a preparation process involving steaming and drying, which enhances its tonifying properties and reduces its purgative effects.

Six Evils: External pathogenic factors that can cause illness and imbalance in the body. They include Wind, Cold, Heat, Dampness, Dryness, and Summer Heat, that invade the body and disrupt its harmony when the immune system is weakened or imbalanced.

Spleen: One of the five organs in Traditional Chinese Medicine, responsible for transforming and transporting food essence, regulating digestion, and supporting immune function.

Stagnation: A state of blocked or impaired energy flow in the body, often leading to symptoms such as pain, discomfort, and imbalance.

Tai Chi: A mind-body practice characterized by slow, flowing movements, deep breathing, and meditation, used to promote relaxation, balance, and overall well-being.

Tao Hong Si Wu Tang: See Four Substance Decoction with Peach Pit

TCM: An abbreviation for Traditional Chinese Medicine, a holistic system of medicine originating in China, encompassing various modalities such as acupuncture, herbal medicine, Qi Gong, and dietary therapy.

Tiao Yuan Duo Zi Fang: See *Rehmannia and Multiseed Decoction*

Urinary System: The bodily system responsible for producing, storing, and eliminating urine, including organs such as the ki1dneys, bladder, and ureters.

Vaginal Steaming: A holistic practice that involves sitting over a pot of herbal steam. It is believed to promote circulation, balance hormones, and alleviate various gynecological issues, although scientific evidence supporting its effectiveness is limited.

Vitality: The state of being strong, healthy, and full of energy.

Warming: A characteristic of certain herbs and foods that promote warmth and circulation in the body, often used to alleviate coldness and stagnation.

Yin: One of the fundamental substances in Traditional Chinese Medicine, representing

Yi Mu Cao (*Leonurus japonicus*): A medicinal herb used in Traditional Chinese Medicine to regulate menstruation, alleviate menstrual pain, and promote uterine health. It is often brewed into teas or decoctions for its therapeutic effects on the female reproductive system.

Zang: The Yin organs, which include the Heart, Liver, Spleen, Lungs, and Kidneys. These organs are considered the primary repositories of Qi (vital energy) and play essential roles in regulating bodily functions and maintaining overall health.

About the Author

Li Mei Chen

Li Mei Chen is a renowned holistic wellness practitioner, blending her expertise in Traditional Chinese Medicine (TCM) with a modern perspective. With a background in acupuncture, herbal medicine, and mindfulness practices, Mei Chen has dedicated her career to helping people harmonize their mind, body, and spirit in the midst of the fast-paced modern world.

Known for her insightful teachings and practical guidance, Li Mei Chen is a respected authority in the field of adapting TCM principles to contemporary lifestyles. Through her work, she inspires people to embrace the wisdom of ancient healing traditions and integrate them seamlessly into their daily lives for sustained well-being.

www.ingramcontent.com/pod-product-compliance
Lightning Source LLC
Chambersburg PA
CBHW071021250726
48653CB00005B/1670